DO107434

Kudos for this Exceptional Book

"As a long-time and extremely satisfied patient, I know that readers will find great interest and value in Dr. Babbush's lucid presentation. His many years of study, research, practice, lecturing, and teaching have made him a truly outstanding leader in this exciting and rapidly growing area of dentistry."

—STANLEY C. GAULT, Retired Chairman and
Chief Executive Officer
Goodyear Tire and Rubber Company and Rubbermaid, Inc.

"This book makes it crystal clear to the reader what implants are all about. It offers hope and remedy for so many who thought they had no alternatives."

—DR. JEROLD GOLDBERG, Dean, School of Dentistry,
Case Western Reserve University

"*As Good as New* lives up to its title. A lay reader can readily grasp the principles and practices of dental implant medicine. The mystery is gone—thanks to the diagnoses, preparations, and remedies explicit in this welcome book."

—LOUIS GROSSMAN, Ph. D.,
Professor Emeritus of Marketing and Management,
Arizona State University

"Down-to-earth is the phrase that best describes this highly informative book by a seasoned dental implant practitioner. The personal anecdotes go beyond human interest. They affirm for anyone who is missing teeth the improvement in the quality of life that implant dentistry has to offer."

—MORTON L. PEREL, D.D.S., M.Sc.D,
Co-Editor, *Journal of Implant Dentistry*

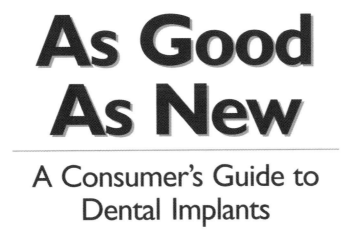

As Good As New

A Consumer's Guide to Dental Implants

Charles A. Babbush, DDS, MScD

The Dental Implant Center Press
LYNDHURST, OHIO

Although the author and publisher have made every effort to ensure the accuracy and completeness of information contained in this book, we assume no responsibility for errors, inaccuracies, omissions, or any inconsistency herein. Any slights of people, places, or organizations are unintentional.

First printing 2004

ISBN 0-9742087-4-4
LCCN 2003107750

ATTENTION CORPORATIONS, UNIVERSITIES, COLLEGES, AND PROFESSIONAL ORGANIZATIONS: Quantity discounts are available on bulk purchases of this book for educational, gift purposes, or as premiums for increasing magazine subscriptions or renewals. Special books or book excerpts can also be created to fit specific needs. For information, please contact The Dental Implant Center Press, 29001 Cedar Rd., #103, Lyndhurst, OH 44124; (440) 995-5500.

Table of Contents

Dedication

I have created and published many works over the course of my 35 years of performing implant-reconstructive procedures. However, none has rallied as many people and entities as *As Good As New*.

I wish to dedicate this project to some of those who made it happen.

- First, to the thousands of patients I have treated over these years.

- Second, to all of my fellow dentists and physicians who have had the confidence to refer patients to me and work as a team to create these successful cases.

- Third, to all the commercial biotech companies that supported, encouraged, and assisted me by developing, creating, and supplying the hardware and software for these cases.

- Last, but certainly not least, to my wonderful, dedicated, and knowledgeable staff: Helen Petsanis, Sherry Greufe, Lori Ruiz-Bueno, Pat Zabukovec, and Ella Mae Shaker. In some instances, they have contributed to all this success for more than 30 years.

Acknowledgments

Many have contributed to the creation of this book.

Writers Jeannette DeWyze and Doris A. Fuller had to be lobbied to assist me in reaching my 10-year goal. But once committed, they completed every deadline on time, as well as offering creative and constructive contributions. It has been my pleasure to work with such a dedicated and professional duo, and I sincerely thank them for their participation. I also thank Ken Sanger and Del Younglas for their knowledgeable and creative preparation of the photographs and diagrams in electronic form.

The success of any health-care procedure as well as that of any doctor can only be measured by the success, confidence, and support of patients. I was overwhelmed by the generosity of my patients who agreed to be interviewed about their experience with dental implants. For their trust and confidence, I sincerely thank James Bondy, Timothy Divito, James Friedman, Jean Friedman, June Goldberg, David Hanbury, Bonnie Hotchkin, Joyce Kammer, Elizabeth Lovsin, Richard S. Miller, Beverly Oppenheim, Joann Platman, Martha Schaffran, Ella Mae Shaker, Jeanette Silber, Warren Silinsky, David Snow, Marscee Wolkis, and Myrtle Watson. All have contributed to the health care and education of the public.

I also am grateful to Marty Dymek, President, Nobel Biocare USA, and Jerry Feeney, Director of Marketing, for their support of this book. Consultant George Smyth has been an inspirational mentor for many years. He contributed substantially to many concepts expressed in this book, and I deeply appreciate his friendship and guidance.

I have called upon several of my dental colleagues to review, critique, and improve the material presented on these pages. These doctors include Fady Faddoul, Michael Powers, and Jeffrey Young. I especially wish to thank Drs. Jay Resnick, Richard Streem, and Evan Tetelman for the significant part they have played in my professional success.

From the commercial side of the implant business, Marty Dymek, John Kay, Bill Ryan, Bob Salvin, Tom Stratton, and Gary Tureski offered invaluable insights into the future, for which I am deeply grateful. Dr. Jack Wimmer, who furnished me with the implants I used to carry out my original research and started me off in this field, has my eternal gratitude for his advice and friendship throughout all these years.

Finally, what a treasure I found when another author introduced me to About Books! There Marilyn Ross, Deb Ellis and Cathy Bowman took the final steps in bringing this book to the public arena, for which they have my heartfelt thanks.

The following companies have supported *As Good As New* with generous grants made as part of their commitment to the health and welfare of the general public:

GenSci Orthobiologics in Irvine, California

**Salvin Dental Specialties
in Charlotte, North Carolina**

**Harvest Technologies Corporation
in Plymouth, Massachusetts**

The Amara Institute in Stillwater, Minnesota

Introduction

Jon was so handsome, he could have worked as a fashion model. At 19, his broad shoulders, strong jaw line, and dark hair drew admiring glances from co-eds on the small Midwestern campus where he was studying government affairs. Jon often zoomed from class to class on his bike, peddling with an effortless grace. It wasn't clumsiness or ineptitude that caused him to crash one blustery fall afternoon—just bad luck, the edge of his wheel catching an unseen concrete edge.

As he plunged downward, Jon's mouth hit the bike's handlebar. And though he was able to get up and dust himself off, Jon immediately realized that the blow had knocked out one of his two front teeth. After a moment of searching, he found the missing incisor and hurried to the campus health center. He felt glum, but he told himself not to worry. "It's the 21st century," he reassured himself. "They can fix these things."

His heart sank when the dentist on duty announced that the ejected tooth probably wouldn't survive re-implantation; too much of the root had broken off. Instead the dentist explained that he could grind down the two healthy teeth on either side of the new gap in Jon's mouth. He would then make a "bridge" containing three teeth. The two caps would be cemented over John's two ground-down incisors, and the middle tooth would fill the hole created by the accident. This was the standard treatment for a lost front tooth, the dentist assured the student. The bridge *would* probably wear out every seven or eight years, and

1

a new one would be required, the dentist acknowledged, a prospect that only further dismayed Jon.

Like Jon, millions of Americans have lost a tooth to injury or disease. And like the college student, many conclude there is no way to return to the state of wholeness they once enjoyed: able to eat any food that appealed to them, unimpeded in their speech, unselfconscious about their appearance, quick to smile.

In this belief, they are mistaken.

Over the past 35 years, I've helped literally thousands of individuals from every walk of life to recover from the disaster of tooth loss. The technological breakthrough that has enabled me and other dentists to do this is the modern dental implant (Figure 0.1).

A dental implant is a small metal post that serves as a substitute for a natural tooth root. Inserted surgically into the jawbone, it provides a stable base upon which an artificial tooth can be anchored. The basic concept is so simple that it occurred to people thousands of years ago. Some even fashioned primitive implants that worked. By the time I entered dental school in 1958, more sophisticated experiments were taking place, but implant dentistry remained a fringe activity. I completed my residency in oral surgery and served in the U.S. Navy for three

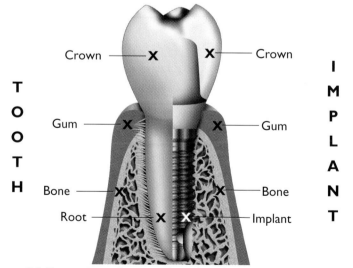

Figure 0.1 Comparison of a natural tooth and crown with that of an implant and crown.

years, including a two-year post in Taiwan. When I returned to enter private practice in the Cleveland area in 1968, I found that more and more articles about implants were showing up in dental trade publications.

I was skeptical. As I scrutinized these reports, I noted with disdain that none appeared to present any scientific evidence that implants could be depended upon to serve patients for years. Implants were a dangerous fad, I suspected, reminiscent of cruder and more primitive times. Then I had a brainstorm. A medical colleague of mine at Mt. Sinai Medical Center in Cleveland, where I was on the teaching faculty, was using geriatric dogs for his research on the relationship between high blood pressure and kidney failure. I asked if he might allow me to replace some of the animals' broken down teeth with implants and study the impact of the implants on the hard and soft tissues of the jaw. My hypothesis was simple: the implants would soon fall out.

My gracious colleague agreed, and in 1968, I undertook my first canine dental surgeries. I anesthetized the animals and extracted two worn and yellow/brown teeth on each side of their lower jaws, replacing them with blade-shaped implants made of Vitallium—an alloy of cobalt, chromium, and molybdenum (Figure 0.2). I let these heal for a couple of weeks, then I fastened onto the implants special gold caps that I wrapped with stainless steel wire. I attached the wire to the adjacent teeth, and covered the gold caps with acrylic—a makeshift tooth with which all the dogs proved able to chew. I waited. And I waited. And I waited some more. (Needless to say, these elderly, ailing animals' mouths weren't the most hygienic oral environments, so I was doubly amazed by what I saw.) Lo and behold, after 18 months, the implants all still appeared to working well!

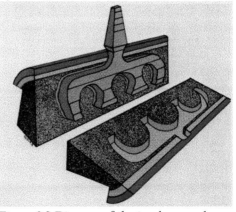

Figure 0.2 Diagram of the jaw bone and gum tissue around a blade-vent implant similar to that used in my original 1968 research.

I was so impressed that within a few months of placing the implants in the dogs, I inserted my very first implant in a patient. Once again, I was astonished by how well my patient was able to function, and I began incorporating implants into my practice of oral surgery. Within two years, I had become a convert. I was convinced that implants would eventually revolutionize dentistry, and I wrote a landmark article about my results, one of the first scientific reports about blade-shaped implants published in the world.

Since that article appeared, the technology of implant dentistry has evolved rapidly. As impressive as implants were in the early 1970s, current designs and materials offer even more extraordinary reliability. Today when my patients ask me how long they can expect their implants to last, I tell them that if I were to place 100 implants the next day (a superhuman task!), 93 to 94 of those implants would still be in place and working well in 10 years. And those implants would have the potential of lasting many more years. I have one patient, for example, who's still being well served by an implant I placed in 1975. She's been so satisfied with it that when one of her other teeth cracked in 2001, the first thing she said was that she wanted another implant.

As the advances in implant technology have taken place, the number of implants placed every year has climbed. Oral surgeons and other dental professionals were expected to perform more than 600,000 implant procedures in 2003 with an annual growth rate projected at 15 percent in the next decade, according to the 1999 Medical Data International Report. That's almost five times as many as took place in 1986.

Still, the number of people receiving implants remains a small fraction of all the people who could benefit from them. Of the 150 million Americans now estimated to be missing one or more teeth, some 35 to 40 million are completely toothless. Sports injuries knock out another two million teeth *every year*, and conditions such as decay and gum disease prompt American dentists to extract another *40 million* or so teeth annually.

Figure 0.3: Tooth Loss in the United States

The number and categories of missing and lost teeth in the United States.

Category	Number
U.S. Population (2000 census)	280 million
Persons missing all teeth	35-40 million
Persons missing one or some teeth	150 million
Tooth extractions annually	40 million
Teeth lost due to accidents annually	2 million

This book is intended to correct the myth that implants still are experimental and undependable. I've tried to use non-technical language to explain to the average reader just what implants can do. The following chapters should make it clear what can be expected from this life-changing therapy.

Statistics compiled by reliable scientific researchers have proven beyond a doubt that implants are safe, effective, and reliable. Yet those statistics don't communicate the human side of what implants do for people. Those stories are so varied that the only way to appreciate their breadth is to hear some of them. For that reason, I've included a Success Story as a little interlude between each chapter.

As Jon, the unfortunate college student, noted at the beginning of this chapter, this is the 21st century. In the wake of inevitable tooth loss, we now DO have the ability to deliver to dental sufferers teeth that are *As Good As New*.

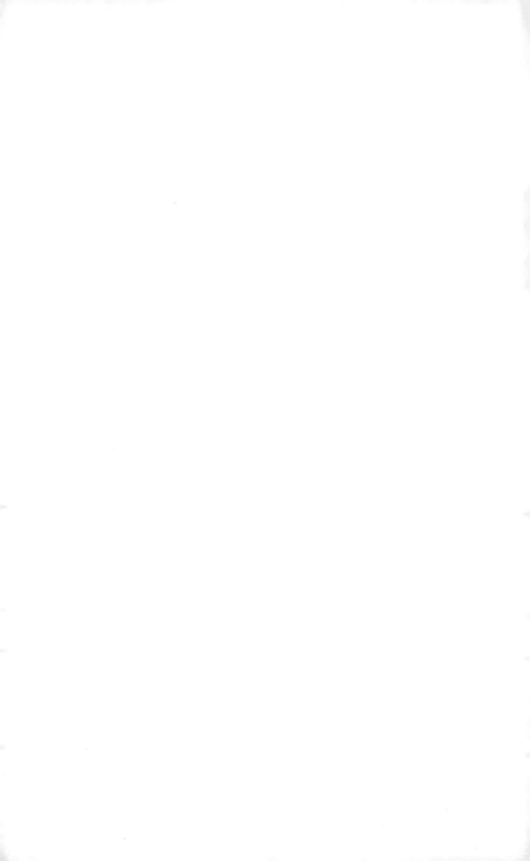

1 *A Profound Breakthrough*

Travel for a moment back in time. It's about 100 years A.D. In Rome, the emperor commands a realm that extends throughout much of the known world.

In the far-flung outpost of Gaul—today's France—a man sits in a dimly lit room and hangs his head in despair. Although he's not yet 30, he already looks old. His mouth hurts, as it has many times before. He can't remember when he had to have his first tooth removed to relieve the suffering it caused him. Over the years, other teeth followed, and now yet another one is tormenting him. Once it is gone, the man fears he will no longer be able to chew the tough meat that provides most of his sustenance. If he cannot keep up his strength, he will die.

The sufferer is willing to attempt an unusual experiment. A friend who is skilled at metal work has offered to make him an iron substitute for the diseased molar. The friend will hammer and fold the metal until the shape resembles the tooth that is failing. Then he will push it into the empty socket. If the iron tooth remains in place, it will help its bearer to survive.

A Long History

Although the details have been obscured with time, anthropologists in 1997 discovered evidence of a story just like this one. The researchers were working in an ancient burial site south of Paris. Along with some pottery, they found a skull containing a wrought iron "tooth." The skull belonged to a young man who lived about 1,900 years ago, carbon dating found. And the operation apparently succeeded. The implant had fused with the jawbone, allowing the man to live with it for at least a year before he died of unrelated causes, the scientists concluded (Figure 1.1).

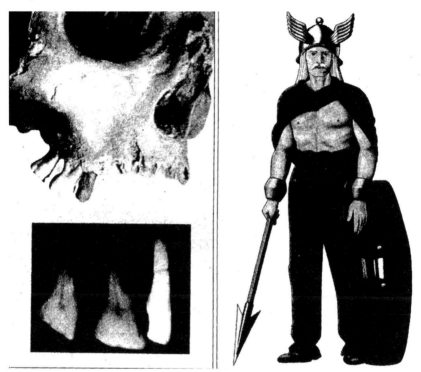

Figure 1.1 Top left, a wrought-iron tooth implant in the upper jaw of an ancient warrior in Gaul. Bottom left, an x-ray of the metal implant. At right is a drawing of a typical warrior of Gaul.

This is the oldest dental implant that has ever been found. But other archeological evidence indicates that humans long before then were searching for solutions to the terrible problem of tooth loss. A fixed bridge featuring four natural human teeth and two carved ivory teeth bound in gold wire was found in Sidon, the chief city of ancient Phoenicia several millennia before the birth of Christ (Figure 1.2). In what is today Italy, Etruscans devised methods of fixing extracted teeth onto gold

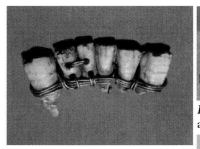

Figure 1.2 Four natural teeth with two ivory teeth bound with gold wire. From the Fourth Century in Phoenicia.

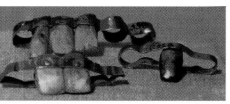

Figure 1.3 The Etruscans used extracted teeth affixed to gold bands to replace missing teeth.

bands like modern bridges (Figure 1.3), while in what is now Honduras, inhabitants used tooth-shaped stones to replace teeth 800 years ago. Fragments of shells have been found in 600-year-old Mayan jaws (Figure 1.4).

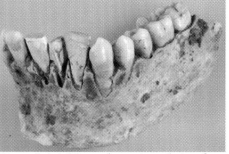

Figure 1.4 A Mayan lower jaw, dating from 600 A.D., with three tooth implants carved from shells.

Most of these primitive attempts at implant dentistry didn't work. Since no one for centuries could figure out how to consistently get tooth substitutes to stay in the bone, dentists throughout most of recorded history concentrated on developing devices that would restore the appearance of normal teeth, if not the full function.

The earliest false teeth date back to Switzerland 500 years ago and were made of ox bones. But this technology was still so primitive by the late 1700s that the first president of the United States couldn't find a well-fitting pair of dentures. George Washington's favorite ones, made of human teeth supported by an ivory base hinged with a spring, tormented him when he talked or ate (Figures 1.5-7).

A number of breakthroughs led to better dentures in the 19th and early 20th centuries, but they remained a poor substitute for natural teeth. By the end of the 1800s, some dentists were ready to take another look at implants. One of the earliest experimenters from this period advocated using dried human teeth. These could come from any source, no matter how old,

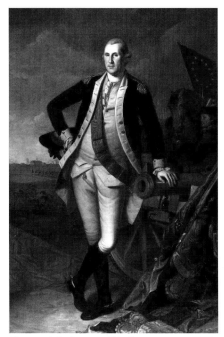

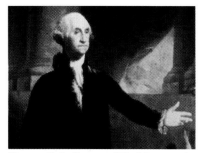

Figure 1.6 George Washington in 1796, after his teeth were extracted and dentures were inserted. His jaw, chin, and lip structure have significantly changed.

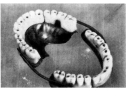

Figure 1.5 George Washington in 1779, before his teeth were extracted.

Figure 1.7 Typical example of false teeth (dentures) made for George Washington. Note the springs connecting the upper and lower dentures. These assisted in keeping the dentures in his mouth.

he insisted. (To prove his point, he implanted a 2000-year-old tooth taken from an Egyptian mummy in one hapless patient!) While many of these tooth-replacements didn't remain in the jaw for long, a small cadre of dentists continued to dabble with various implant designs and materials ranging from porcelain to lead to rubber to cattle teeth.

A Metal that the Human Body Could Love

The crucial breakthrough finally came in the 1950s, with the identification of an ideal implant material: titanium. A Swedish medical doctor made this discovery. Per-Ingvar Brånemark had been studying the way bone heals. As part of that research, he had inserted a titanium chamber into the leg of a rabbit because it allowed him to study the animal's bone marrow under a microscope. When he completed his observations several months later, he tried to remove the expensive piece of equipment and found to his annoyance that he couldn't get it out. Bone had grown into the titanium, apparently fusing with it.

It wasn't until some time later that the significance of this emerged: here was a material that the body not only did *not* reject but that bone seemed to love. Titanium also did not appear to irritate skin or other soft tissue. Perhaps medical and dental implants should be made out of titanium, Brånemark's research team began to think. Over the next ten years, they conducted extensive studies of the biomolecular processes that occur when titanium is placed in living tissue. By 1965, they treated their first patient, a 34-year-old man who had been born with a deformed chin and jaw that made it impossible for him to speak or eat normally. Four post-shaped titanium implants were implanted in his jaw and allowed to heal. Later a set of false teeth was connected to them.

The surgery transformed the patient's life, and the implants are still working well to this day. Brånemark then went on to refine the techniques for placing dental implants. By 1977, he had won the endorsement of Swedish health authorities and begun training other Swedish dental experts

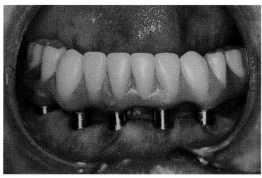

Figure 1.8 Brånemark implant and fixed denture restoration of a lower jaw, as done in the early 1980s.

to follow his example. He presented his 15 years of meticulous animal and human research to all the leading North American dental researchers at a meeting in 1982. The presentation finally established implants as a mainstream treatment option (Figure 1.8).

Advances that have taken place since then have been phenomenal; today implants routinely restore natural function to millions of people who have lost some or all of their teeth. The appearance of implants has also improved dramatically. Today, when a front tooth is lost, it is possible to create an implant-

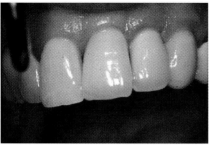

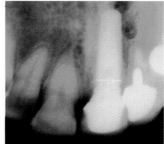

Figure 1.9A This patient's left central crown, attached to a single implant, is virtually indistinguishable from the natural teeth.

Figure 1.9B The x-ray of the implant in place in the front upper jaw.

supported replacement that is indistinguishable from the original tooth (Figures 1.9A,B). Patients with advanced gum disease and bone deterioration may not regain quite that level of cosmetic perfection. However, they can expect implants to match or improve upon their appearance compared to wearing a denture or a bridge. And of course, the implants feel like real teeth. As one patient who had lost all but six of her own teeth before replacing them with implants says, "I feel like they grew there."

What's the Alternative?

Despite the proven benefits of implants, the majority of the millions of Americans who are missing teeth are still replacing

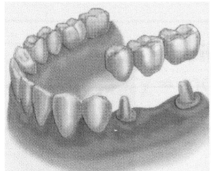

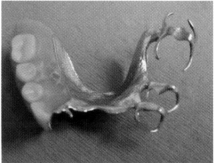

Figure 1.10A Traditionally, a single missing tooth has been replaced with a three-unit bridge. This treatment requires the teeth on either side of the space to be shaved down to receive the crowns. Suspended between them is the dummy tooth (pontic).

Figure 1.10B This removable partial denture replaces four missing teeth in the upper jaw. It covers the roof of the mouth and has hooks that clasp it to the remaining natural teeth.

them with either bridges or partial dentures (Figures 1.10A,B). Both options can have serious drawbacks.

Every bridge has to be anchored to something. To secure the bridge, the dentist must create anchor teeth, grinding them down just as when a tooth is being covered with a crown. In many cases, perfectly good teeth are sacrificed.

Full or partial dentures carry with them unintended consequences that are usually even more unpleasant than the compromise of two good teeth for a bridge. That's because dentures rest upon the gum tissue; they don't stimulate the underlying bone in the same way a natural tooth root or a dental implant does. A natural tooth or an implant stimulates the bone, which the bone needs to remain healthy. In the absence of such stimulus, the bone begins to shrink.

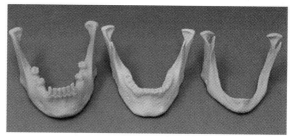

Figure 1.11 These models illustrate progressive bone loss in the lower jaw. At left is a normal jaw with the teeth present. In the middle is a jaw seen shortly after the loss of the teeth. On the right is the jaw 15 years after tooth removal, when 60 percent of the bone has been lost.

This phenomenon plagues astronauts in zero gravity. It affects paralysis victims. And it dooms even the best-designed dentures (Figure 1.11).

The shrinkage in the jawbone changes the denture-wearer's appearance. When the bone in the back of the jaws deteriorates, the front teeth often flare out and the corners of the mouth droop. As the bone continues to melt away, muscles typically shift out of their normal position. Wrinkles appear, and the appearance of the cheeks becomes distorted. Ultimately, the loss of jaw height can cause the nose to point downward and the chin to curl up, creating a witch-like appearance. As the lips lose their support, they become flattened, further accentuating the appearance of age (Figures 1.12A-D and 1.13A-H).

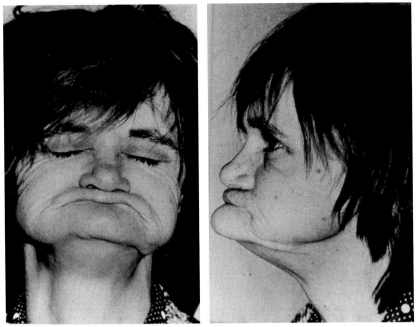

Figures 1.12A,B A front and side view of a 41-year-old patient's face eight years after losing her teeth. Severe jaw shrinkage has occurred. Note the prominence of the chin and nose and collapse of the lip structures, which accentuates the appearance of age.

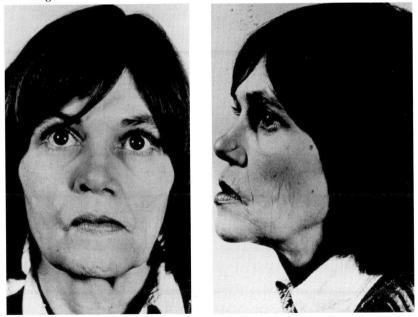

Figures 1.12C,D A front and side view of the same patient's face after implant reconstruction of the lower jaw with new upper and lower dentures.

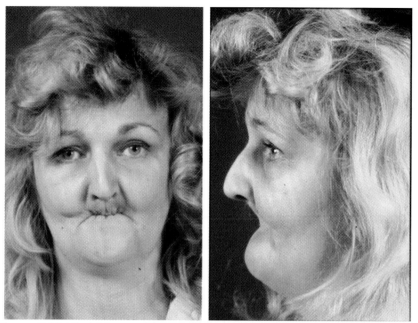

Figures 1.13A,B A 33-year-old patient who lost all her teeth as a teenager to decay and gum/bone infections. The advanced jaw shrinkage has severely compromised her appearance.

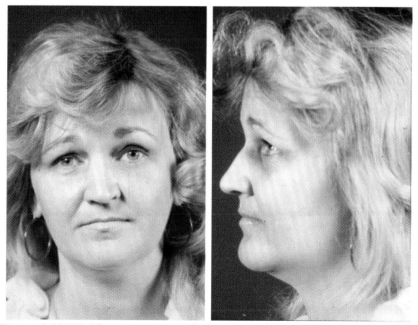

Figures 1.13C,D The same patient after receiving lower-jaw implants which are supporting new dentures. She also received a new upper denture.

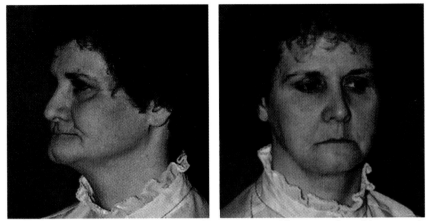

Figures 1.13E,F This patient lost all of her upper and lower teeth and has a moderate amount of subsequent jaw shrinkage.

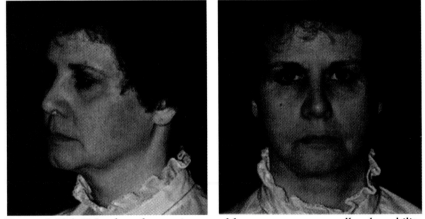

Figures 1.13G,H Implant therapy improved her appearance as well as her ability to function.

In addition to the disastrous cosmetic consequences, most people have trouble with the way their dentures fit as their bone melts away. Over time, less and less muscle and bone remain to hold the dentures in place. Nerves within the lower jawbone get closer and closer to the surface. Some individuals wind up suffering pain with every bite they take. For others, the poor fit of their dentures may become an overwhelming problem. That's what happened to James Bondy, who underwent successful implant treatment for his lower jaw in the mid-1970s

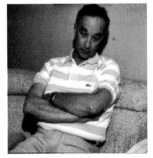

Figure 1.14A

but continued to struggle for years with an upper denture that would not stay in position. Eventually, he became so frustrated that he gave up wearing it, in spite of the difficulties it created at every meal.

Hordes of people experience the sort of difficulties that plagued James. Like him, many simply give up. They resign themselves to being toothless, accepting the discomfort, inconvenience, and social stigma that accompany that state. Their self-esteem often plummets. Men and women alike may undergo personality changes or sink into a chronic depression (Figures 1.14A,B).

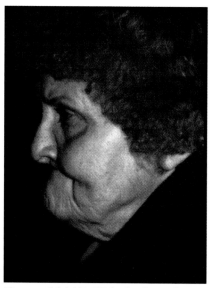

Figures 1.14A,B With the loss of teeth and resulting jaw shrinkage comes difficulty biting, chewing, and digesting food, along with increased pain, depression, and emotional problems. Overall quality of life is often impaired.

The Hurdles

Given that implants have the power to dispel all the agony that so often accompanies toothlessness, why don't more people choose them?

Cost is certainly one factor, but it's one that must be evaluated in light of how crucial well-functioning teeth are to every person's survival. Teeth are equipment used for the vital business of eating, several times every single day. People who lose their teeth no longer face death from starvation as the desperate young Gaul did, but without a stable, comfortable, substitute, nutrition is almost certain to deteriorate.

At the same time, millions of Americans every year undergo cosmetic surgery procedures that in many cases cost as much or more than implants. They pay for these surgeries in order to correct "problems" that are far less vital to their health and well-being than those caused by missing teeth. Likewise, millions of people take advantage of laser surgery to correct their vision, even though most insurance policies don't cover this procedure. When something is important enough, people usually find a way to pay for it.

Another reason why more people don't choose implants is that all too many don't realize they have this option. Perhaps their dentists haven't kept up to date with the fantastic developments that the past two decades have brought. Perhaps those dentists have resisted implants because they see them as being some sort of economic threat to their own practices.

This has finally begun to change. Both the National Institutes of Health and the American Dental Association have declared that implants are now the standard of care. This means they are an accepted technique and can no longer be considered experimental. And word about implants is finally reaching patients.

James, the patient who gave up on his ill-fitting dentures, eventually chose to have seven implants placed in his upper jaw. Because he had lost so much bone there, he had to undergo a lengthy bone-grafting procedure in conjunction with the implant placements. Looking back five years after his final surgery was completed, he recalled that he had experienced some physical discomfort, "but it wasn't too bad." And with full function and a normal appearance restored, he added, "I could never imagine going without my teeth again, that's for sure!"

David Snow

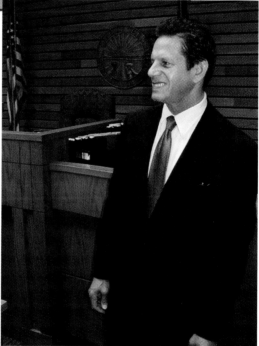

Many patients are devastated at the thought of losing their teeth. As a doctor, I find it tremendously gratifying to see their joy and satisfaction when they regain their quality of life with implants, as David did.

David Snow remembers the chill that gripped him when he heard the grim prognosis: his periodontal disease was so advanced that infection was raging in his mouth. All his teeth would have to be extracted.

"I wanted to run out of the office; go to another country. I wanted to go to another planet! *You're taking my teeth? I don't think so!*" Snow says he felt like someone was telling him his right arm had to come off—then trying to comfort him with assurances that it could be replaced. He wanted to scream in response: *You can't replace my right arm! I'm a pitcher.* In actual-

ity, Snow is a criminal defense attorney in Cleveland. His liveli-
hood depends upon his ability to speak, and the thought of doing
anything to jeopardize that ability terrified him.

Somehow, a lifetime of dental problems had failed to prepare him for this ultimatum. Now 53, Snow recalls making trips
to the dentist as a young child. "There were lots and lots of fillings." Crowns later replaced most of the fillings. At 15, Snow
also was diagnosed with diabetes, a serious medical condition
that typically increases the risk of tooth decay and gum disease.

By the time he was in his 40s, all his remaining lower teeth
had fractured at the gum line. Essentially all that remained of
them was the roots. The situation in his upper jaw was little
better, with chipped crowns and missing teeth intermingling.
Still Snow says he never imagined losing all his teeth. One day
he elected to have some minor cosmetic surgery, and he was
taken aback by a question posed to him by the plastic surgeon. "He asked me why I didn't do something to fix my teeth," Snow recalls. "Well, when somebody makes a comment like that, you have to think about what he's say-ing."

> **David Snow:**
> *I can't tell you how fast I started eating corn and apples. I hadn't eaten apples in ten years. There are things the doctors understand about how your body works that no layman would understand. What I've gotten cannot be overstated. Forget about eclipses! Or seeing a comet for the first time in your life. I haven't gotten new teeth; I've gotten a whole new existence.*

Snow consulted one im-
plant specialist and had three
implants placed in the lower
jaw. But he never got around
to having teeth attached to
these implants, a lapse on which he blames his busy schedule.
"By the time I got to Dr. Babbush's office, my dental problems
had gotten so bad that none of my teeth could be saved."

Despite his initial panicked reaction to his prognosis, Snow
soon was calmly evaluating his options. He was told that he could
have all the remaining teeth extracted, wait several months for
the sockets to heal, then undergo implant surgery (wearing dentures during the healing periods.) Or he could choose a surgery

in which he would receive both final and temporary implants that would enable him to leave the operating room with functional interim teeth in his mouth. The cost of this option would be higher because of the additional implants, and the initial surgery would be a complex one.

Snow chose the latter course. In addition to his diabetes, he'd developed several other major medical problems, and an active life had caused him to break more bones over the years than he could remember. The prospect of a long surgery didn't faze him.

He arrived as scheduled at the outpatient surgery center at six o'clock one morning in April of 2000. The surgery lasted close to seven hours. In the course of it, all Snow's teeth and the three previous implants that were never restored and subsequently failed were removed. They were replaced with 17 standard implants and 11 smaller provisional ones that would support the temporary teeth while the bone fused with the standard implants and healed. His damaged jawbone was built up with grafting material, and platelet-rich plasma made from his own blood also was used to speed up the healing process and improve the quality of the bone and the gum tissue.

When Snow thinks back on how he felt upon awakening from the anesthesia, he says he has little memory of any discomfort. Nonetheless, the implants were a big change. Since he hadn't had any fixed teeth for years, his surgery "wasn't like getting new teeth," he attests. "It was like getting a new mouth. And getting a new mouth is more significant than getting a new arm. You get a new mouth, and you have to learn to talk again." Assured that his brain would adjust to all the changes—that he would soon stop biting the inside of his cheek and speak as fluently as ever—"I wanted to say, 'How?' But I just shut up because there are things the doctors understand about how your body works that no layman would understand."

Sure enough, in the days that followed, Snow overcame his initial difficulties. "I went to work just a couple of days after the surgery. I believe that, like a quarterback, when you tear an ACL, you still have to play. You don't even tell anyone you have a broken knee. You just play. Because the game is much more important than your little pain." As the days passed, his speech got clearer and clearer, and he began to feel a sense of confidence about his new mouth that amazed him.

"I can't tell you how fast I started eating corn and apples," he exclaims. "I hadn't eaten apples in ten years." Associates at the courthouse commented on his new, improved appearance, and his self-confidence began to soar. He still faced a long waiting period and numerous appointments with the restorative dentist. But by the time Snow was ready to receive his permanent teeth in January of 2002, he'd become so fond of his temporary teeth that he almost didn't want to give them up.

Today he can't find enough superlatives to describe the permanent teeth he received in place of the temporary ones. Taking care of them has been "so easy that a boy could do it," he says. Because his surgical and restorative work was so extensive, all the work cost more than $50,000, but Snow declares, "It's been worth $50,000 *every day!*"

He says getting implants was one of the most profound experiences of his life. His new mouth has made him feel like the Six-Million Dollar Man. It has given him a smile Tom Cruise would envy, he says.

"What I've gotten cannot be overstated. Forget about eclipses! Or seeing a comet for the first time in your life. I haven't just gotten new teeth; I've gotten a whole new existence."

2 Are Implants for Me?

If anyone had predicted Joyce Kammer would need dental implants, "I would have told them they were crazy," she says today. Everyone in her family had good, strong teeth, and Joyce's father, a dentist, coached his children in the fundamentals of oral hygiene. "Teeth were very important in our house, and they were taken care of all the time," Joyce recalls.

But one day in her late 20s, Joyce was involved in a serious car accident. "I slammed my whole face against a steering wheel," she recalls. One by one, her teeth underwent root-canal treatment and were capped. Over the years, problems developed with the caps, and she lost the underlying teeth. To replace them, her dentist made removable partial bridges for her, but they never fit well. "I was very uncomfortable wearing them, and I was told that I was losing bone. Everything led me to the point where I felt the only thing I could do was implants."

As Joyce points out, tooth loss "happens to the best of us. It could happen to anyone." Millions of people lose their ongoing battles with decay and periodontal disease; tens of millions don't get regular professional care. And as Joyce learned, accidental injuries can also claim teeth from the healthiest mouths.

While every person might at some point lose a tooth, it is *not* true that every individual who is missing teeth should have implants. Implants are not a panacea. They work best when placed in a strong foundation of bone and nourished with a healthy blood supply. Other dental, medical, psychological, developmental, and financial considerations can also make someone a less-than-ideal implant candidate.

This chapter looks at some of the things to be considered when determining whether implants are for you.

Dental Considerations

The first and foremost of the considerations are those involving the conditions that exist in the patient's mouth.

Bone and gums

Implants achieve their tremendous strength and permanence because something almost miraculous happens after the implant has been placed in the jaw. Over time, the bone grows into the microscopic irregularities in the implant surface until, to the naked eye, the metal and bone appear to have fused together into a single entity. Dentists call this process "osseointegration." (The word comes from "osseo," meaning bone, and "integrate," meaning to unite.)

For osseointegration to succeed, the bone must firmly grip the implant when it is placed. Enough bone must be present to support the implant completely. The stronger and denser the bone, the better. But human jawbone varies tremendously—both in its quantity and quality. Years of wearing dentures as well as other factors can weaken and wear down the bone until what remains cannot support an implant.

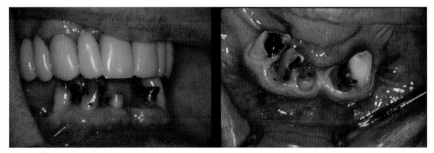

Figures 2.1 Multiple fractured and decayed teeth, as well as infected gums.

Over the past 20 years, dentists have developed dependable procedures for transforming weak and inadequate jawbone into a good foundation for implants. In the same fashion, when the amount of gum tissue is inadequate or when gingivitis or periodontal disease are present, these conditions must be addressed, and the health of the soft tissue must be restored (Figure 2.1).

Bruxism

The ancient Greeks were familiar with teeth clenching and grinding since they had a word for it: *brychein* (literally, gnashing of teeth). Most people tap, clench, and grind their teeth upon occasion, but some folks—perhaps as many as one out of four—do it so often and so excessively that it damages their teeth (Figure 2.2).

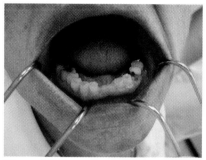

Most often this occurs during sleep. This "nocturnal bruxism" can apply astonishing levels of force to the teeth,

Figure 2.2 Excessive wear, or abrasion, of the patient's lower teeth.

gums, and jaw joints—up to ten times the amount generated by normal chewing. Upon a newly placed implant, that kind of force can be catastrophic, making osseointegration impossible.

If you clench and grind your teeth excessively, that doesn't mean you're not a candidate for implants. Protective action such as wearing a night guard may be necessary for a favorable result, however.

Adequate access

In order to place the vast majority of dental implants, the dentist must be able to use a drill and other tools inside the patient's mouth. Sometimes trauma or treatment for tumors or other disease can prevent patients from opening their mouths wide enough to permit this.

Once again, solutions to this problem usually can be found. An implant of an alternative design, such as a mandibular staple implant or a transmandibular implant (TMI), can be placed by creating an incision underneath the chin and drilling upward through the bone. Either of these implants is then placed through the prepared sites.

Medical Considerations

Many physical conditions have an impact on how well dental implants will succeed. As the art and science of implant dentistry and general medicine have evolved over the past few decades, fewer and fewer medical problems remain *absolute* contraindications for implants. But some absolute contraindications still exist. Other conditions might be called *relative* contraindications—likely to cause trouble if they're ignored but not a problem if they're dealt with properly.

Let's take a look at each in turn.

Absolute contraindications include:

Pregnancy

Anesthesia, x-rays, and pain medication all pose some level of risk to the unborn child. For this reason, pregnant women should postpone implant treatment until after delivering their babies.

Advanced dermatological disease

A number of disorders can affect the mucous membranes, gums, and skin. (Examples of some of these soft tissue defects include erythema multiforme, lichen planus, lupus erythematosus, and pemphigus.) Patients with even mild cases of these diseases may have flare-ups including ulcerations and severe pain: imagine a mouth full of canker sores or blisters, and you can understand why such people are usually not good implant candidates.

Malignant disease

Radiation, surgery, or chemotherapy treatments for cancer impose tremendous stress on the immune system. For that reason, it's best to defer undergoing any implant procedures until such treatments have been successfully completed.

Once the person has recovered from the cancer therapy, success with implants can usually be expected. One exception is the individual who has received primary or secondary radiation directly to the jaws. Such treatment often badly damages the blood supply to the jawbone. Drilling into the bone to place implants may further disturb the blood supply, and the bone may begin to deteriorate as a result.

An alternative for people in this category is to undergo an extensive series of treatments in a hyperbaric oxygen chamber. Exposure to the oxygen-rich atmosphere in the chamber—both before and after implant surgery—increases the blood supply to the jaw. This auxiliary treatment, while costly and time-consuming, has been shown to make implant treatment both feasible and successful.

Human beings are living longer than ever. As they age, many develop diseases that can be controlled well enough to allow them to enjoy their lives. Most such diseases fall into the category of relative contraindications for implants. If untreated, these and other disorders can reduce the chances that the implant will osseointegrate and function well. But when they are addressed properly, most patients can feel confident that dental implants will work well.

Common medical conditions in this relative contraindication category include:

Smoking-related health issues

Smoking a single cigarette reduces the speed at which blood flows to the fingers by more than 40 percent for up to an hour. The restricted blood flow impairs the body's ability to heal. Smoking even as few as five cigarettes a day appears to have negative effects.

The good news is if you can stop smoking for two or more weeks before having implant surgery and continue to abstain from cigarettes for a minimum of eight more weeks afterward, your implants are just as likely to be successful as those placed in non-smokers. (Of course, this may also be an ideal time to stop smoking totally.) In contrast, smokers who don't change their behavior have a much poorer prognosis. Studies have shown that implants placed in smokers are up to three times more likely to fail.

Diabetes

This complex metabolic disorder can cause complications throughout the whole body. In the mouth, it is associated with higher rates of tooth decay and gum disease, along with dryness, an increased incidence of infection, and other changes. Healing after surgery appears to occur more slowly.

When patients control their diabetes with diet, insulin, or other means, studies have shown that they can enjoy as much success with implants as non-diabetic patients. Only for the so-called "brittle diabetic" is the picture less rosy. This term refers to those individuals who have trouble maintaining a good degree of health and hygiene, both physical and oral. Their insulin requirement continually fluctuates and is difficult or impossible to control. For such people, a good outcome is less likely.

Hemophilia

Not so long ago, this bleeding disorder was considered to be an absolute contraindication for implants. Today, however, such patients can be treated before surgery with a substance known as cryoprecipitate. It supplies the factor that's missing from their blood and permits it to clot normally, so surgery can be performed safely.

Epilepsy

Many epileptics are now able to control their convulsions with medication. They live a normal life. For anyone who falls within this category, implant surgery should not present extraordinary risks. Uncontrolled epileptic seizures, on the other hand, could endanger the patient during surgery and anesthesia. Moreover, these seizures may cause the victim to bite down with a force that can damage dental implants.

It's worth noting that the anti-seizure drug, Dilantin, in some people can cause an enlargement or overgrowth of the gum tissue around the teeth or implant abutments. When this does occur, it is readily treatable.

Impaired movement

Strokes, severe arthritis, amputation, and paralysis all reduce a person's ability to perform the steps necessary to keep his or her mouth and implants clean (see Chapter 8).
In the absence of good oral hygiene, implants are likely to fail. However, this obstacle may be overcome if family members or other caregivers are able to perform cleaning routines for the patient.

Other medical disorders

A host of additional medical conditions may either affect the course of implant treatment or be affected by it. These include heart arrhythmias, angina, rheumatic heart disease, chronic bronchitis, emphysema, ulcers, liver dysfunction, kidney disease, and more. Virtually all are relative contraindications, as is the presence of other artificial replacements in the patient's body. The conscientious practitioner will discuss any such condition with the patient's physician. If he or she approves the patient for implant surgery and anesthesia, every effort should be made to control the condition as well as possible.

If you're trying to decide whether implants are for you, keep in mind the impact of such medical disorders. After ten years, 93 out of 100 implants placed will still be functioning well. If the same 100 implants were placed in heavy smokers who also had high blood pressure and diabetes, roughly 85 to 90 of the implants could be expected to work well after five years; after ten years, the number might be as low as 75 to 80 implants. If you're a smoker who has high blood pressure and diabetes, and you don't keep those conditions under control, are the odds good enough for you? That's a decision each individual patient must make.

The Impact of Age

At the upper end of the spectrum, medical science has demonstrated conclusively that you're never too old to have implants. In the absence of other medical problems, age alone carries no negative impacts.

Children, however, are a different story. The problem with placing implants in youngsters is that their jaws have not finished developing. As the jaw grows, the implants may move out of position, causing a variety of problems.

At what age is a child old enough to have a missing tooth replaced with an implant? This varies from one individual to the next, but most girls stop growing by 14 to 16. Most boys get to their maximum size a bit later, at 16 to 21. The height of the parents and older siblings, as well as the presence of all the permanent teeth, can be a helpful guide in determining if full growth has been achieved. In the rare case of the child with congenitally missing teeth, implants may be placed under a modified protocol before the child is fully grown.

Until it has, the missing tooth can be replaced with a retainer-type partial called a "flipper," a bonded tooth, or some other temporary solution. This is important not only for esthetic and functional purposes, but also to maintain the space and prevent other teeth from shifting into it.

Psychological Limitations

The mind can have a powerful effect on the health of the body. This truism applies to dental implants.

If you're contemplating getting implants, you should be aware of potential psychological issues. You should ask:

Are my expectations realistic?

If you can't be comfortable with anything less than a guarantee of 100 percent success, implants probably aren't the right choice for you. Virtually no medical or dental procedure can offer that kind of guarantee. Dental implants rank among the most dependably successful artificial replacements, but things sometimes don't go as expected. When that happens, a variety of measures can usually solve the problem.

Patients should think about what they hope to achieve by getting implants. Sometimes people harbor unrealistic esthetic expectations. The 70-year-old man who walks into the dental office secretly hoping that a few implants will restore his appearance to what it was at 30 is setting himself up for certain disappointment. So is the woman who announces to the doctor that she's ashamed by the appearance of her teeth, when in reality, she's more distraught about the fact that her last child has just graduated from college and her husband is having an affair. She's hoping subconsciously that by changing her looks, she can save her marriage.

People who are seeking solutions to bigger life problems need to look beyond the dental implant.

Do I have a hidden fear of some aspect of the implant surgery?

Some people do. Some are afraid of needles, for example. Nowadays, however, this phobia can be easily overcome with anti-anxiety medication, psychological support or counseling, or a combination of these.

Other individuals unconsciously equate tooth loss with the end of femininity and masculinity. A woman might have only two teeth remaining in her mouth. They might be broken down and decayed; they might look horrible. Yet the thought of having them extracted may well make the woman's blood run cold—not because she fears pain or feels so attached to these particular teeth, but rather because in her mind, toothlessness will strip her of her femininity. For men, it may threaten a loss of virility. Other individuals, like David Snow, experience tooth extraction as being like the amputation of a limb.

Once again, such fears, while very real, are not insurmountable. Talking about them can go a long way to quelling them, and post-surgical medication also sometimes can help patients deal with feelings of depression. Moreover, such individuals usually find that implants restore their sense of normalcy. It's not uncommon for patients to reach a point, a year or two after surgery, when they declare that they feel like they have their own teeth back in their mouths.

Financial Considerations

In answering the question of whether implants are for you, one final area deserves some discussion: cost.

The first and most basic question—how much do implants cost?—has no simple answer. Do you need one single implant or an entire mouthful? Do you have enough bone or do you need grafting? Where do you live? Costs of treatment can vary significantly from one part of the country to another.

With that caveat, the following figures, obtained from a survey conducted in 2001, offer some guidance for what you can expect your dentist to charge.

Figure 2.3: Typical Implant Treatment Costs

The average cost of several different types of implant rehabilitation in the United States.

Type of implant treatment	Average cost	Range of fees
Single tooth	$ 3,182	$2,035 - $ 5,500
Three teeth	$ 8,483	$6,300 - $12,750
Clip-bar overdenture supported by five implants	$14,445	$9,450 - $24,000

Figures 2.4A-C illustrate each of these treatment options.

Although some insurers will reimburse patients for implants that become necessary as a result of a trauma or tumor, most dental insurance policies do not cover the majority of implant procedures. The argument can be made that this is shortsighted. When the *total* costs associated with traditional dentures or bridges are compared to the cost of implants, implants may turn out to be less expensive.

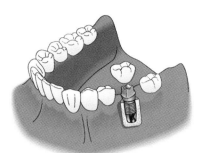

Figure 2.4A
A single implant and crown.

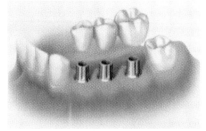

Figure 2.4B Three implants and crowns.

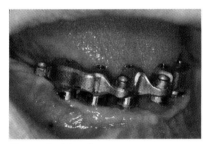

Figure 2.4C A lower jaw restoration with five implants and a connector bar. An overdenture clips onto the bar.

The Institute for Dental Implant Awareness has calculated, for example, that if a single, implant-supported crown costs between $2,500 and $4,000, the alternative of a tooth-supported bridge over the course of 20 years will be approximately $6,000 to $7,000. The larger figure includes the costs of grinding down the two teeth on either side of the missing tooth, replacing the bridge at least once, and repairing the bone loss that is certain to occur over the course of two decades.

Hopefully, as more and more consumers need and demand treatment with implants, dental insurance companies will take a longer view. In the meantime, every individual must weigh the costs and benefits. The first office visit should greatly help to clarify these. The next chapter looks in depth at what typically happens on that appointment.

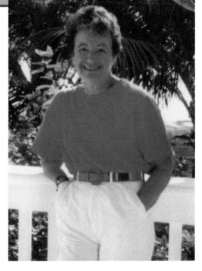

Typically, patients have lots of time to reflect on whether to have implants, but not all do. In the case of my patient Beverly, the decision was forced on her in an instant.

Who could guess that the road to dental implants might begin in Africa?

Certainly Beverly Oppenheim wasn't thinking about her teeth when she set off for Kenya in January of 2002. "We had been planning a trip there for 18 months," Beverly recalls. "My husband and I had been to Africa four times before, and we wanted my daughter and her husband to experience it."

The two couples met in London, where they celebrated the beginning of their adventure by attending an evening performance of *The Lion King.* The next day, they made the long journey to Amboseli National Park, renowned for its abundant animal life and stunning views of Mt. Kilimanjaro. Their first full day in the park began auspiciously. "We had a wonderful morning and saw all kinds of animals," Beverly says.

During a second game run in the afternoon, rains freshened the dry landscape. Upon their return, Beverly and her daughter set off for the lodge bathing facilities, a walk that took them over slabs of marble covering a pathway edged with pointed cones of lava rock. Beverly was just commenting about the perfection of her accommodations—in an opulently furnished tent with a king-size bed and a stunning view of some nearby elephants—when she slipped on the wet stone under foot.

Beverly Oppenheim:

After the implant surgery, I took one pain pill because Dr. Babbush insisted I do so, but I was never in pain. It was like magic. They feel just like my own teeth and they look great.

"I went down, and my upper jaw hit the lava rock." She gathered herself together and realized that the blow had dislodged several teeth. "They came out in my hand."

Her forehead also was bleeding profusely. Beverly's daughter, a nurse, bandaged her wounds but expressed concerned that her mother might have suffered a concussion.

The next morning, a flying medical service landed a small plane at the park and transported the injured American to a modern medical complex in Nairobi. "It was wonderful!" Beverly exclaims. "The dentists had computers and x-rays, and they treated me very well." She already knew the bad news: that several teeth were broken beyond repair. But no sign of any concussion could be detected.

A plastic surgeon on the staff expertly sewed the cut on her forehead, and the next morning, Beverly and her husband headed back to London, after insisting that their daughter and son-in-law continue on with their African safari.

"I was not in pain," Beverly recalls of her stopover in England. "My husband and I checked into a hotel near the airport, took the underground train into the city, toured the portrait museum, and had dinner at our favorite restaurant, where I ate the Dover sole." The next day they continued their trip home and hurried to the offices of their trusted family dentist.

Never before had Beverly, 71, lost any teeth. She'd heard a little about implants but had no idea what was involved in implant treatment. Still, she didn't hesitate when her dentist referred her to me. Within days, she underwent surgery in which her broken tooth roots were extracted and four implants were placed into the sockets. Bone-grafting material and platelet-rich plasma were applied to help promote the healing at the site and ensure its strength.

After the implant surgery, "I took one pain pill because Dr. Babbush insisted I do so," Beverly says. "But I was never in pain. It was like magic!" Over the next five months, she wore a temporary bridge that was designed to keep pressure off the healing implants. "Also I couldn't eat anything hard. That was the only difficult part, and I did fine with it. It wasn't that bad."

In June of 2002, Beverly's family dentist removed the temporary bridge and cemented her final teeth into position. "They feel just like my own teeth, and they look great," she testifies. She adds that the accident has in no way dampened her enthusiasm for travel. Just four months after receiving her final prosthesis, she and her husband enjoyed a lengthy trip to Prague, Budapest, and Vienna. "My husband was in the export/import business, so travel is in our blood. The accident in Africa was the first time anything has ever happened to either of us." Thanks to the high-quality medical care and the ease of the implant treatment she received, she says the accident is already a fast-fading memory.

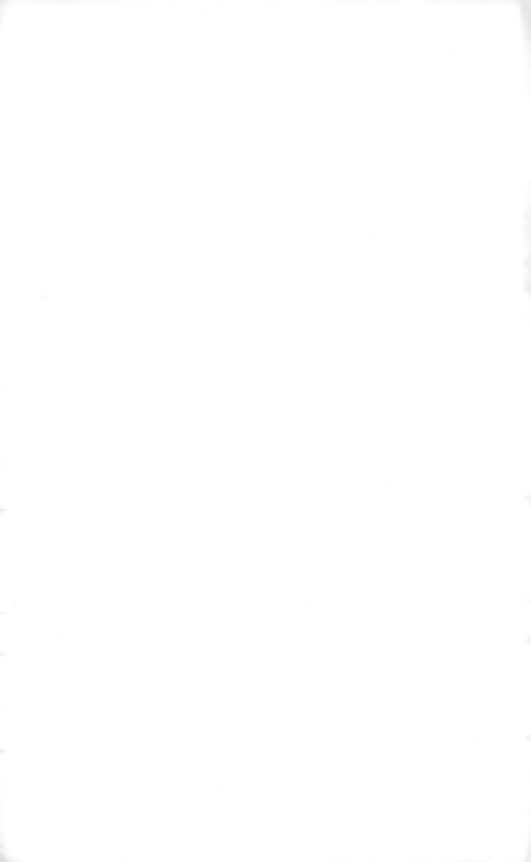

3 *How Do I Choose an Implant Doctor?*

Americans are the greatest consumers on earth. We shop more, buy more, and spend more per person than citizens anywhere else. In the process, we have become expert at sorting through competing brands of everything from corn flakes to cars to find the products that suit us best. We ask friends and relatives about their experiences and recommendations, and we consult consumer magazines, buying guides, and online bulletin boards to get detailed information. For major purchases, we may visit several retail outlets and interview multiple sales representatives before making a final choice (Figure 3.1).

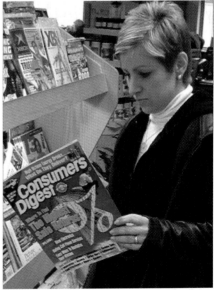

Figure 3.1 Many consumers need advice when looking for a new product.

If you are considering dental implants, selecting the right implant doctor demands just as much attention.

With proper diagnosis, treatment, and post-treatment maintenance, dental implants can be part of your body for many,

many years—very possibly for the rest of your life. Unlike the salesman who sells you a refrigerator or new tires for the car, you will see your implant dentist for years of routine follow-up. Taking the time and effort to find the right doctor is a small initial investment for a big, long-term pay-off.

But where do you start? Unlike the washing machine or the computer that you can turn on in a local store or read about in *Consumer Reports*, you don't get to "test drive" your implant doctor or look up his/her rating in a buyer's guide. It's easy to feel so stumped that picking a name from the Yellow Pages begins to look good.

It shouldn't. By bringing the same skills and thoughtfulness to finding the right implant doctor that you do to finding the right vehicle, your chances of a long and happy relationship with *both* your implants and your implant doctor will be greatly enhanced.

A Little Background First

Before you start hunting for the right implant doctor, it's helpful to understand a bit about the dental profession and where implants fit into it.

Elsewhere in the world, a single trained implant doctor often provides complete treatment from diagnosis through surgery to final restoration. This arrangement occurs in the United States, too, but far more common is a "team" approach in which the implant surgery and restoration are handled by different doctors.

The doctors who place and restore implants or belong to an implant team are not "specialists" in the way that oral surgeons, prosthodontists, or periodontists are. They don't have to meet specific educational requirements or certification requirements in order to practice implant dentistry. Historically, continuing-education classes have provided this education. More recently, some dental schools have begun offering or requiring undergraduate students to study and/or be trained in the basic technology and techniques of implant dentistry, but this is not universal.

Implant treatment may someday evolve into a specialty with its own dental residency programs and certification. If the history of the profession is any guide, however, implant therapy will continue to be offered by specially trained dentists who arrive in the implant field from a variety of starting points. These include:

General dentistry

An estimated 131,000 practicing dentists in the United States have completed dental school, with some of those following those studies with a one-year general practice residency that did not focus on any specialty. Not all general dentists work with dental implants. Of those who do, most concentrate on restoring the implants with new crowns, bridges, and overdentures after implants have been placed by a surgical specialist. A smaller number of general dentists handle both surgery and restoration.

Oral and maxillofacial surgery

The next largest group of dental professionals, numbering around 6,500, are dentists who finished dental school and then underwent a lengthy residency in surgical technique. Oral and maxillofacial surgeons were the first dentists to acquire training in the placement of implants and in supplementary surgical procedures such as soft tissue and bone grafting. Few oral surgeons also restore implants.

Periodontics

These 5,000 surgical specialists treat the gum tissue that surrounds the teeth and other hard and soft tissues of the mouth. Some place implants and perform supplementary surgeries. Like oral surgeons, few restore implants.

Prosthodontics

Numbering a little more than 3,000, these dentists specialize in making crowns, bridges, dentures, and other forms of replacement teeth. Most are skilled in restoring dental implants, but few place them.

Typically, you won't have to choose your whole implant team. Once you find a surgeon or a restorative dentist you want to work with, chances are good that h/she will refer you to the companion professional with whom h/she routinely works.

The rest of the team

Your doctors may be the co-captains of the implant team, but its success requires the active participation of several other players:

- the dental laboratory, which fabricates the metal framework and the new teeth that it holds

- the dental assistant, who provides you with instructions and information, answers your questions, and assists the doctor at chairside during various procedures (Figure 3.2)

- the hygienist, who provides professional maintenance and cleaning of your teeth and implants over their long life (Figure 3.3)

- an implant coordinator, who is designated specifically to coordinate implant schedules, administration, and team members and to answer questions from patients—not every practice has a staff member in this role (Figure 3.4)

- you, the patient, the single most important team member once treatment is complete

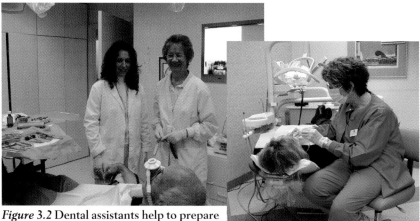

Figure 3.2 Dental assistants help to prepare the patient for a procedure.

Figure 3.3 A dental hygienist is an important part of the implant team.

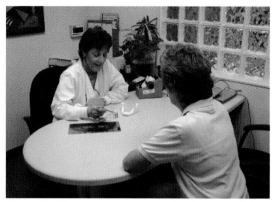

The ongoing health of your bones, gum tissues, and implants depends upon your habits of daily brushing, flossing, and other maintenance and your keeping of professional follow-up appointments.

Figure 3.4 In many practices, an implant coordinator helps to explain procedures to prospective patients.

Identifying Candidate Doctors

Knowing what the completed team looks like is the equivalent of identifying the features you need in your new car. Once you know, you're ready to begin looking for the right one.

Like many patients, you may find an implant doctor within the course of other dental care you are already receiving. Perhaps you bring up the topic of implant treatment with your family dentist, and it turns out h/she has an active implant restoration practice and knows several excellent oral surgeons who can place the implants. Or you've been undergoing treatment for gum disease with a periodontist you like and trust. When you decide to replace some of your teeth with implants, you have an established relationship with a doctor who can handle your surgery and refer you to a good restorative dentist to round out your team.

If the dental professionals within your existing circle of health-care providers don't provide implant services and are not a source of referral for you, here are several other strategies for finding good candidate doctors.

Casual word of mouth

The first and perhaps best way to identify candidates is to ask for personal recommendations from friends, relatives, neighbors, co-workers, and others you trust. Although individual experiences differ and personal recommendations are not infallible, the positive recommendations of existing happy patients who have no reason to be anything but completely frank are always an excellent starting point (Figure 3.5).

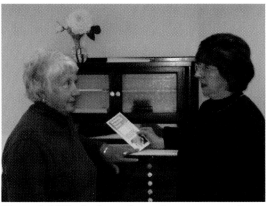

Figure **3.5** Word of mouth can be a strong endorsement.

Professional word of mouth

Your family physician or a medical specialist you know and trust may be familiar with the work and reputations of the dental providers in your communities. Friends or acquaintances who work in the dental field often will have "inside" insights that can help you develop a list of possible doctors.

Dental associations

Professional associations such as the American Association of Oral and Maxillofacial Surgeons, International College of Oral Implants, the Academy of Osseointegration, and similar groups include doctors who provide implant services. Many of these organizations maintain a referral base for consumers. A complete list of these organizations with their contact information is listed in Appendix B.

What's in a Letter?
DDS or DMD? Does the title make a difference?

In a word: No. "DDS" stands for "Doctor of Dental Surgery." "DMD" represents "Doctor of Dental Medicine." The education and degrees are the same, only the letters are different. Most dental schools in the United States award a DDS degree, although some still confer a DMD. Dentists in Canada, Great Britain, and other countries use other titles and designations to signify the same information.

The Next Step

Referrals are a good beginning. Good research needs to follow. This may include:

Calling the prospective practice

Call and say you've been given the doctor's name because you are considering dental implants. Ask if an information packet can be mailed to you. Excellent implant literature is readily available to every implant practitioner. If the one you call doesn't have any or requires you to come to the office for an appointment before you can see it, you may want to move on (Figure 3.6).

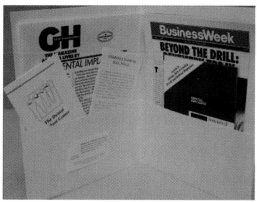

Figure 3.6 Written information is an important educational tool.

It may also be useful to ask for a short biography of the doctor. A fact sheet such as this might answer questions you would otherwise have to wait to ask.

Scheduling a consultation

A consultation is the perfect time for you to ask about the doctor's qualifications and distinctions. Because certification is not required to practice implant dentistry, the training and experience of your doctor candidate are both relevant and important. In other words, you want to know the doctor's track record.

Questions you might ask include:

• How many years have you been placing/restoring dental implants?

• How many implants have you placed/restored?

- What portion of your practice do implant procedures make up?
- Do you track the success rate of your implant cases? If so, how many of the implants you place/restore are still in place and working 10 years later? Twenty years?
- What kind of continuing education courses in implant dentistry do you take or have you taken?
- Do you belong to any professional implant organizations?
- Do you do research, write, or teach about implants?

In most offices, there is a fee for the consultation appointment, but the cost is typically quite small relative to the total cost of implant treatment. Because policies vary among doctors, you may want to ask about the doctor's fee policy before scheduling the appointment. If your prospect can't answer questions such as these, or if h/she becomes testy when questioned, this again may be a signal for you to move on. Your relationship with your implant doctor will be a long one. Over that period, a variety of questions may arise that you want answered. Finding a doctor who responds to reasonable questions readily and candidly is essential.

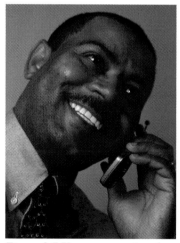

Figure 3.7 Your prospective doctor may put you in contact with a patient who has already been treated.

Talking with someone the doctor has treated already

Upon request, your prospective doctor may put you in contact with a patient h/she has already treated. Usually, measures will be taken to protect the previous patient's privacy and yours. You should remember that it's inevitable that you will be referred to a happy patient, not one who has doubts about the doctor. Even so, the current patient is another source of "word of mouth" information and can provide you with a patient's-eye view of the doctor you're considering that nobody else can offer you (Figure 3.7).

Making the Right Choice

In all but the smallest communities, you will be able to choose from among a number of implant doctors for your surgical procedures, your restoration, or both. Taking the steps outlined above should lead you to one or more candidates capable of providing you with successful dental implant treatment. However, before making your final decision, don't overlook one last critical factor: your instincts.

It is possible to find a doctor with the best credentials in the world, the highest level of experience, the greatest number of cases, and the most complete record of dealing with every possible complication or contingency—and still not have found the right doctor. If you don't feel comfortable with a clinician you're considering, if your confidence isn't inspired, you need to keep looking.

At the foundation of every good, lasting doctor-patient relationship is trust. Only when you have found that will you know you've found the doctor for you.

ADA Recommendations

The American Dental Association suggests that any time you are choosing a dentist, you ask yourself these questions:

- *Is the doctor's appointment schedule convenient for you?*
- *Is the office easy to get to from your home or job?*
- *Does the office appear to be clean, neat, and orderly?*
- *Were your medical and dental histories recorded and placed in a permanent file?*
- *Does the dentist explain techniques that will help you prevent dental health problems?*
- *Are special arrangements made for handling emergencies outside of office hours?*
- *Is information provided about fees and payment plans before treatment is scheduled?*

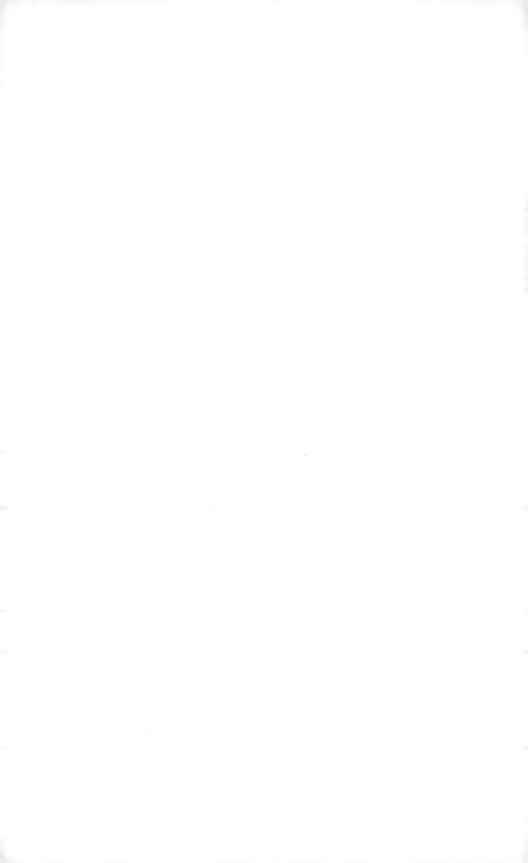

Richard S. Miller

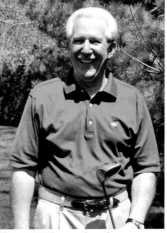

Most of my patients come to me by referral from another doctor or a previous patient. Richard was exceptional —in more ways than one.

Richard Miller's natural teeth nearly cost him his life.

Richard was born with a congenital cardiac problem that created an area in the heart where bacteria can collect. When this happens, a life-threatening infection of the heart's lining can develop.

People with this type of heart problem are required to take antibiotics before any kind of surgical procedure or dental treatment, and Richard was no exception. He was in his early forties when he went to the dentist for a routine cleaning on a day when he'd forgotten to take his antibiotics. He confessed his oversight, but the cleaning was done anyway. A few days later, his temperature begin to rise. Eventually, it reached 105 degrees, and he grew too weak to stand or walk. By the time he checked into a hospital, he was gravely ill with subacute bacterial endocarditis—infection of the heart. For two weeks, he fought for his life.

It was 32 days before he left the hospital. "I almost died," he says.

Though by far the most devastating health episode of his life, the endocarditis was far from the first dental crisis Richard had faced.

I grew up in a children's home and never learned basic dental hygiene as a child. By the time I was approaching my teens, I had a lot of problems with my teeth and gums. I must have been 12 or 13 when I finally went to the dentist, and he drilled into a nerve. It was such a harrowing experience—I didn't even have Novocain—that I didn't go back."

Neglect and fear teamed up to undercut the young man's dental health. Within years of his painful dental mishap, permanent teeth were rotting in place. Often, he pulled them out with his own fingers. By his twenties, the shape of his mouth was beginning to change from all his losses. "I was becoming deformed—literally" by the gaps, he says.

At last, Richard went back to the dentist. Over the next several years, teeth were pulled, teeth were capped. Bridges were used to fill voids where teeth once grew. The bridges required the sacrifice of adjacent teeth to support them, but eventually these supporting teeth began to break down because of the gum disease. Root canals followed. His regime of professional care and routine maintenance was meticulous, but no matter what he tried, nothing could return him to anything approaching normal dental health.

"The bridges and dentures lasted, but they weren't permanent, and they were never right. I couldn't chew. I couldn't swallow. I'd bite into a sandwich and choke on the food," he

> **Richard S. Miller:**
>
> *I can't tell you how much dental implants improved my feeling about how I looked and spoke. I can eat, I can talk, I can whistle.*
>
> *I have a confidence I didn't have before. My teeth are no longer held in by wires or clips or glue. They are screwed into place. Even my facial structure has improved because of the bone grafting. I simply couldn't put a value on them, they are beyond price.*

recalls. A successful businessman, "I didn't want to smile. I did things to protect myself. Because of the periodontal disease, I had chronic bad breath. Quirky things would happen. I was washing my bridge once before going to a bar mitzvah, and it broke in half while I was cleaning it. I had to stay home."

It was during this period of his life that Richard and I met and began our long and close friendship. Eventually Richard brought up the subject of implants.

"I'd heard about implants and found the idea of having all my teeth pulled and replaced appealing. Chuck urged me to save the teeth that could be saved, and that's the approach I took for a long time. But after endocarditis followed a routine cleaning, I didn't want to be at risk any more. I went to Chuck and said, 'Can we do the implants now?' "

Following thorough diagnostics, a plan was developed that called for placing seven implants to hold a removable full overdenture in Richard's upper jaw and one implant each on the right and left rear of the lower jaw to help secure fixed lower bridges. Bone grafting would be done to restore some of the jawbone Richard had lost over the years.

The two of us have jointly celebrated our birthdays—which are four days apart—for 20 years. As it turned out, Richard's implant surgery was scheduled on my birthday. He arranged for the operating room personnel to sing "Happy Birthday," and then we started the procedure. As a survivor of bacterial endocarditis, Richard is more vulnerable to heart infection than he was before his life-threatening episode. As a result, his implant surgery was performed in a hospital, and he stayed for the night afterward. With appropriate surgical preparation and procedures, there were no complications. "It wasn't even painful," Richard says of his surgery.

That was in 1990. Richard says his life was never the same after implant surgery. It was better. Dramatically better.

"I can't tell you how much dental implants improved my feeling about how I looked and spoke," he says. "I can eat, I can talk, I can whistle. I have a confidence I didn't have before. My teeth are no longer held in by wires or clips or glue. They are screwed securely into place. Even my facial structure has improved because of the bone grafting."

Richard Miller lost his teeth and underlying bone to early neglect. Implants and bone grafting have given them back to him.

"I simply couldn't put a value on them," Richard says. "They are beyond price."

4 The Initial Office Visit

Every implant case begins with a story.

Maybe it's a story like that of Timothy Divito, an active 16-year-old who lost his upper right incisor in an athletic accident at a high school track meet. Already in the grip of teenage self-consciousness, Timothy was embarrassed by his removable "flipper" replacement tooth and wanted something that looked and felt more natural.

Or perhaps it's a story like 73-year-old Warren Selinsky's. Warren was on his second set of upper dentures in ten years when he made his first implant appointment. He wanted to eat and smile again without feeling his teeth shift in his mouth.

Possibly, the story is similar to James Friedman's. A 46-year-old with periodontal disease and tooth decay that required the removal of many of his natural teeth, James considered his options and decided the best one for him was dental implants.

You have a story too. Whether it parallels one of these or not, your implant dentist wants to hear it. The initial visit is your chance to tell it.

What Happens at the Initial Visit

The initial office visit to your implant doctor typically lasts 30-40 minutes and has two main goals:

1. To give the doctor the personal, medical, and dental history needed to decide whether you are a candidate for implants and;

2. To give you, the patient, the practical and financial information you need to decide whether implants are for you.

A great deal of information is discussed in this meeting, and important decisions are made on the basis of it. Some implant candidates find it helpful to take notes to refresh their recollections later. Others bring a husband/wife or close friend to the appointment for the same reason.

The information elicited and exchanged in the initial visit falls into five general categories:

- the reasons you are seeking treatment
- what you want from your treatment
- your medical history
- your dental history
- a comprehensive oral exam, which may include some preliminary diagnostic procedures such as taking impressions and/or x-rays

You can plan for your initial implant visit by thinking about each of these categories as the appointment approaches.

Reasons for Seeking Treatment

Patients arrive at their initial consultation appointment for a host of reasons, as the stories that opened this chapter only begin to illustrate. The first thing your doctor will want to learn are your specific needs, wants, and desires. He will probably also ask what motivated you to call for this appointment.

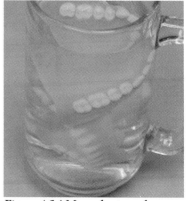

Figure 4.1A Many dentures become so unsatisfactory they are left in a glass of water on the nightstand.

For some people, these motives are primarily functional. They have lost their ability to bite and chew their food, to have security when they smile, or to be free of pain. Perhaps the bones of their jaws have shrunken so severely because of tooth loss that their dentures only fit for a few months after each remake or reline before they again become loose and uncomfortable (Figures 4.1A,B). In many cases, their

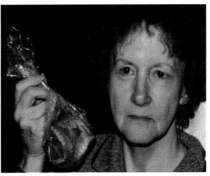

Figure 4.1B Some patients suffer through numerous partial and full dentures in an attempt to obtain a successful result. However, due to the lack of a good foundation of jawbone, satisfactory function with dentures becomes an impossible goal.

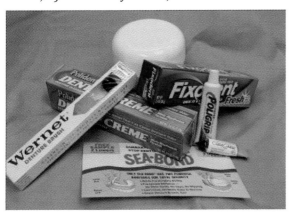

Figure 4.2 Many patients turn to the wide variety of denture adhesive pastes, glues, and pads to hold their dentures in their mouth more securely.

teeth only feel snug when they use denture adhesives and/ or powders (Figures 4.2). Maybe they cannot wear dentures at all, a situation that often leads to secondary problems such as poor nutrition.

For other patients, the chief complaint is cosmetic. They are self-conscious about smiling with a denture in place. They feel embarrassed by the appearance of damaged or unhealthy natural teeth. They have unsightly gaps where teeth were lost and never replaced. They want to feel better about the way they look.

Needs, wants, and desires are highly individual. Patients with jobs that rarely bring them into contact with the public may be concerned primarily with how their teeth work. Those working in the spotlight may be motivated chiefly by concerns about appearance. A concert trumpeter won't be able to play her instrument reliably if her teeth aren't secure in her mouth; she may be seeking a solution to a problem that affects her career.

The more clearly you can identify and describe *all* the reasons you are seeking dental implant treatment, the more likely it is that your doctor will develop a successful treatment plan with you. The patient who finds it difficult *and* painful to chew food, for example, very likely has different functional issues that need to be addressed than the patient who merely finds it difficult to chew.

Closely related to your reason for investigating implant treatment is the history of your condition and the factors that created the problem you have. Did you lose a tooth to an accident or to a tumor? Have you lost one tooth, some teeth, or a whole mouthful of teeth? Are you currently wearing a dental prosthesis—a partial or full denture, bridge, or flipper—and, if so, how is it working for you? What do you like and dislike about it? Have you replaced any of your lost teeth already and been unhappy with the replacements?

The dentist will pay particular attention during this part of the evaluation to the circumstances that contributed to the situation at hand. If medical conditions contributed to tooth loss, these may need to be eliminated or brought under control before implant treatment can proceed. If poor dental hygiene, a lack of routine dental care, or failure to address dental problems in a timely fashion was involved, your current habits of dental self-care will need to be addressed. That's because, like natural teeth, implants require daily maintenance.

Medical History

As the previous chapter explained, medical conditions can and do affect your candidacy for dental implants and the treatment plan that is developed for you. This is why a medical assessment is always part of the initial consultation.

This assessment typically will consist of three parts:

- a health questionnaire that you fill out

- discussion with the doctor of any health issues identified in the questionnaire, and
- an assessment of vital signs, such as blood pressure and pulse.

Typically, you will be asked to fill out the health form while waiting for your first appointment to begin. This questionnaire will ask about past illnesses, injuries, and surgeries and about special circumstances, such as whether you are taking medications, suffer from drug and/or other allergies, are pregnant, and/or whether you smoke.

At some point during your visit, the doctor will review your medical history with you. If you haven't undergone a complete medical check-up in several years or if your answers reveal health issues that could possibly complicate or affect the success of your implant treatment, you may be asked to see your medical doctor before implant treatment begins. Additional testing, such as blood work or urinalysis, may be recommended. The doctor may also take your vital signs—blood pressure, pulse, and respiration—and note them in your chart.

Your incentives for treatment will also be evaluated from a psychological standpoint. If the doctor finds your expectations of treatment unrealistic or detects unreasonable fears, s/he will try to help you adjust your outlook and expectations.

When the medical assessment is complete, the doctor will determine your level of surgical risk along the lines described in the previous chapter. If the risks are high, treatment will be modified accordingly. For example, if you are high-risk because of heart disease or high blood pressure, your doctor may schedule implant surgery for the outpatient surgical center or a hospital instead of the dental office.

In most cases, there will be nothing to indicate you shouldn't move on to the next step: evaluation of your dental status.

Dental Examination

Your doctor has already learned about your dental history. Once s/he's reviewed your medical history, s/he'll evaluate the current status of your teeth, jawbone, gums, and other surrounding tissues and anatomy.

No matter how healthy the rest of your body may be, your mouth must be in a good state of repair before implant treatment can begin, or the results will be jeopardized. If your gums are unhealthy, they will have to be treated. If you have teeth that are failing, they will need to be treated and/or removed. A good program of routine, daily home care will need to be established in addition to a pattern of routine professional check-ups.

The dental evaluation begins with an evaluation of your entire face. The doctor will look at its symmetry and proportion and at the influence of any tooth loss on your appearance. When teeth are lost and the jawbone shrinks, the lower third of the face can appear to collapse, causing the chin point or the nose point to look more prominent than they should. The mobility of your jaw—your ability to move it forward and back and to "open wide"—will be checked.

Next, the interior of your mouth will be assessed. If you wear dentures, you will be asked to remove them. If a friend or relative is accompanying you to the appointment and you feel uncomfortable being seen without your dentures, your companion will understand if you ask for privacy at this point. If you alert the dentist prior to the appointment, s/he can help you by asking this person to step out of the consulting room for a few minutes or taking you to another examination room for this portion of your visit.

Now your dentist will look at your remaining teeth to evaluate their condition and assess how the upper and lower teeth relate to one another when you bite. S/he will check the so-called "soft tissues" of your mouth: the inner cheeks and inner aspect of the lips, the floor of your mouth, the tongue, hard and soft palates, and gums. S/he will look for inflammation or signs of abnormality—a tumor, lesions—and at overall oral health. All these factors must be considered in developing your treatment plan.

In most practices, a panorex x-ray will also be taken during the first appointment. Unlike the periapical x-rays taken with the little film packets placed inside your mouth to provide information about two or three teeth at a time, a panorex is taken from outside your mouth and provides a panoramic view of the inside of your mouth and all the nearby anatomy. It shows all your teeth in one picture, including their relationships to one

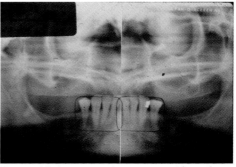

Figure 4.3 A panoramic x-ray provides a large overall view. In contrast, periapical x-rays show a smaller, more restricted area of the mouth (that of the outlined area).

another and to the surrounding structures such as nasal and sinus cavities (Figure 4.3).

Photographs may also be taken of your face and mouth, inside and out, at this appointment or a future one. These become a visual record used by the implant team for reference throughout and at the end of treatment.

Education

The education that takes place during the initial office visit is a two-way street. The doctor learns about you, and you learn about implant treatment. At some point during the initial consultation—perhaps while the x-ray

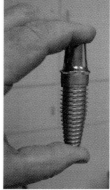

Figure 4.4A A large replica of an implant can be used to assist the orientation and education of a patient during the consultation appointment.

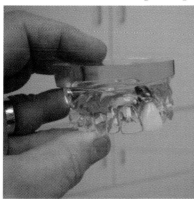

Figure 4.4B Model of a single implant and crown.

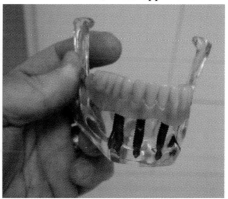

Figure 4.4C Model of four implants and a connector bar with a clip-on overdenture.

is being developed—it's possible you will be shown an educational video sharing general information about implants and implant treatment. The dentist may show you models of implants and actual implants so you can see how they look (Figures 4.4A-C). Before you leave the office, you may be given a packet of informative literature.

The dentist will also give you feedback throughout the meeting on what s/he's learning about your candidacy for implant treatment. Once s/he has finished the medical and dental evaluations and reviewed your x-ray, s/he will be ready to talk to you about the topic that brought you to the office in the first place: your own treatment options based on the combination of needs, wants, and desires you expressed early in the appointment and the information gathered during its course.

Treatment Planning

Although you have probably already considered and possibly dismissed other options, your dentist may start by reviewing non-surgical alternatives for replacing your lost or failing teeth. These typically include (Figure 4.5):

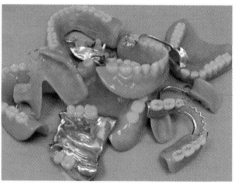

Figure 4.5 Flippers, removable partial dentures, and full dentures.

- Full upper and/or lower removable dentures, if no natural teeth remain

- Partial upper and/or lower removable dentures, if some natural teeth remain

- A bridge cemented permanently in place and involving one or many teeth

- A "flipper," which is a removable appliance with one to several replacement teeth attached to a plate much like a dental retainer

Having covered the non-implant alternatives, the clinician will go on to describe an implant treatment plan that the doctor's experience and your specific situation indicates will best suit your needs, health, and dental status. This plan will address:

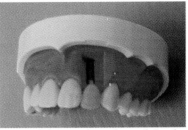

Figure 4.6 A single endosteal (in the bone) implant.

- How many implants you are likely to need

- What kind of implants will be used (Figures 4.6, 4.7, 4.8)

- Approximately where these implants will be located in your jaw(s)

- Any preparatory procedures that might be required to correct situations that could otherwise disqualify you from receiving implants—including measures such as bone grafts or grafts of gum tissue

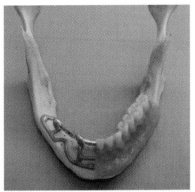

Figure 4.7 A subperiosteal (on the bone) implant.

- What you can expect from treatment in terms of appointment time, anesthesia, medications, follow-up visits, healing, recovery, discomfort, and total duration

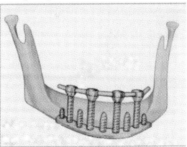

Figure 4.8 A transosteal (through the bone) implant.

- Surgical and other risks associated with dental implant treatment—including failure of the implants, which are vulnerable to poor maintenance, health factors, and other issues just as your natural teeth were

- The maintenance routines your implants will require once treatment is complete

- The cost of treatment, payment schedules, other financial requirements, and insurance considerations

In some dental offices, a computer program will be used to provide you with an image of what your face and mouth may look like once your implants are in place and restored.

On occasion, it's not possible for the doctor to present a complete treatment plan at the initial appointment because more diagnostic information is needed. These procedures can include:

- Occlusal films – x-rays that show your upper and lower jaw widths and alignments

- Lateral cephalometric images (a precise x-ray of the side of your upper and lower jaw that provides an exact side or lateral image)—exact measurements to be used in your surgery and restoration can be made from this x-ray

- Computed tomographic (CT) scan—a three-dimensional image which provides more detailed information about the quantity and quality of your jawbones, such as the distance between potential implant sites and vital structures such as your sinus cavities in the upper jaw and the nerve canal in the lower jaw

If one or more of these diagnostic procedures are needed, they will be completed before your treatment plan is developed in order to make sure the plan is completely appropriate.

Decision Time

On the other hand, if your medical and dental status qualify you as a candidate for treatment, if no further diagnostics are needed, if implants appear appropriate for you after all this information is exchanged, a preliminary treatment plan will be developed during the appointment and some diagnostic procedures are likely to be performed.

A mold of your teeth may be taken. This mold will be used to pour a plaster model of your remaining teeth, your jawbone level, the relationship of your teeth to one another, and the relationship of your jaws to one another. All the team members—who may include the laboratory technician as well as your doctors—will refer to this model as your treatment

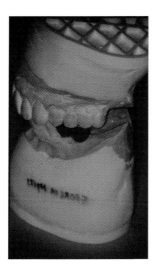
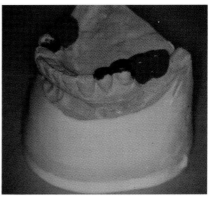

Figures 4.9A,B The blue and red wax on this "study model" shows the doctor the projected implant/tooth result.

progresses. It will also be used to develop what's called a "diagnostic waxup," which is a projected replica of what your teeth and jaws will look like when the treatment is finished (Figures 4.9A,B).

The dentist will present you with some choices that you will make before treatment begins (see *Decisions You Will Make*). You should be given plenty of time to consider these options and make all your decisions thoughtfully. A good implant doctor is one who understands that implant treatment is a significant dental and financial undertaking. S/he appreciates that you need time to absorb all the information the initial meeting produces and to consider your treatment plan. S/he knows you will want to talk to your spouse or other family members or friends. S/he may be able to provide you with referrals and urge you to interview some of these people to hear firsthand about their experience with implants before you proceed with your own. Conferring with your general dentist, prosthodontist, or other team members before making your final decision may also be warranted unless you are dealing with an urgent situation, such as a fractured or painful tooth.

Pressure to make an immediate decision and set your surgical appointment is unwarranted. If you experience this, you should consider another practice for your treatment.

Whether your decision must await the findings of additional diagnostic measures or you and your doctor say goodbye at the end of the initial consultation with all the information you both need, you are likely to meet with your doctor one more time to review the finalized details of your implant treatment plan. Your doctor may also send you a letter once you have scheduled your implant treatment. This letter will note your surgical appointment date, time, and location and restate the key information you've covered in your meetings such as the number and type of implants to be placed, a description of how your individual surgery will be performed, a review of what you can expect after your surgery, any other procedures that will be undertaken as part of your treatment, and your fee and payment schedule. You will want to retain one copy for your files and return the doctor's copy with your signature.

At some point after you make the choice to undergo implant treatment and before your surgical appointment, you will be given an Informed Consent Form to sign and return to the dental office. It is important to read this form closely. Consent for any health-related procedure can only be informed if you've received and considered all the relevant information.

Whether you leave the initial office visit with a referral for more diagnostics, with instructions for stabilizing an uncertain medical or dental condition, or with a preliminary treatment plan, you are on your way—one step closer to an implant solution for the loss of your teeth, your smile, and your normal dental functioning.

Decisions You Will Make

Although your implant doctor or team will make the clinical decisions required for your treatment, in most cases, the following decisions will be made by you with your doctor's agreement.

Types of prosthesis

The prosthesis is the substitute tooth or teeth fabricated to restore the dental implant. It is also called the "restoration." It can replace one or more teeth.

When all the teeth in an upper or lower jaw or both are replaced, this may create options that you will discuss with your doctor, including:

- Fixed prosthesis—the new teeth are fitted to a metal frame, and the frame is permanently connected to the implant abutments. This type of restoration can be removed only by the dentist (Figures 4.10A,B).

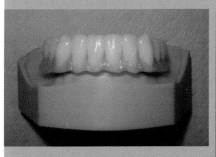 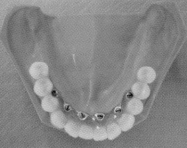

Figures 4.10A,B Model of a lower-jaw implant reconstruction. These implants are screwed into place and are not normally removed.

- Fixed-removable prosthesis—the teeth are set into a removable device such as a bridge that you can place and remove at your discretion for cleaning. The bridge snaps over a bar that joins the implants together; the bar cannot be removed by the patient (Figure 4.11).

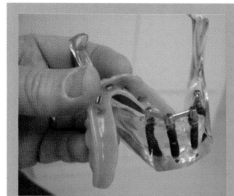

Figure 4.11 This fixed removable prosthesis can be removed by the patient. Lower jaw implants support it.

• Fixed partial prosthesis—when only one or a few teeth are being replaced, a partial prosthesis will be placed. If a single tooth is being replaced, this restoration is typically cemented permanently in the mouth in much the same way a crown is secured over a natural tooth. When more than one tooth is being replaced, you may be able to choose between a fixed or removable denture, just as patients replacing all their teeth do.

Considerations in selecting a prosthesis include:

• Cleaning—a removable prosthesis is somewhat easier to clean and maintain than a fixed prosthesis and is stable when in place

• Stability—a fixed prosthesis may provide even greater stability for chewing than a fixed-removable prosthesis but can only be removed by the doctor

• Cost—a removable restoration in some cases can be secured with fewer implants than a fixed restoration that replaces the same number of teeth (these cases may result in a lower total treatment cost)

Anesthesia

The choice of anesthesia is a function of patient preference, medical history, and the length and complexity of your case. When medical risk factors or conditions are present, your selection of an anesthetic may require consultation and clearance from your physician. Three types of anesthesia are typically available to dental implant patients: local anesthetic, twilight sedation and general anesthesia.

Location

Unless medical history or conditions or the complexity of your implant treatment dictates where your implant surgery is performed, you may choose the location you prefer in conjunction with your doctor. Implant surgery takes place in one of three kinds of facilities: private dental office or clinic, outpatient surgical center (ambulatory or walk-in surgery center) or a hospital, which often requires with an overnight stay.

The rest of the team

If the dentist you see at your initial appointment is a member of an implant team, s/he will refer you to another member for the portion of the care that is provided by another team member. If s/he's a restorative dentist, you will be referred to the surgeon; if s/he's the surgeon, you will be referred to the restorative dentist.

If you are being treated in a large urban area, it is possible that the doctor you first consult works with more than one team of implant doctors within the larger area. When this is the case, you may be offered a choice of team members for your total treatment. Location and convenience are factors you may want to consider in exercising this choice.

If you will be undergoing preparatory procedures such as gum or bone grafting, you will be asked to make additional decisions related to these. Those options will be discussed in Chapter 6.

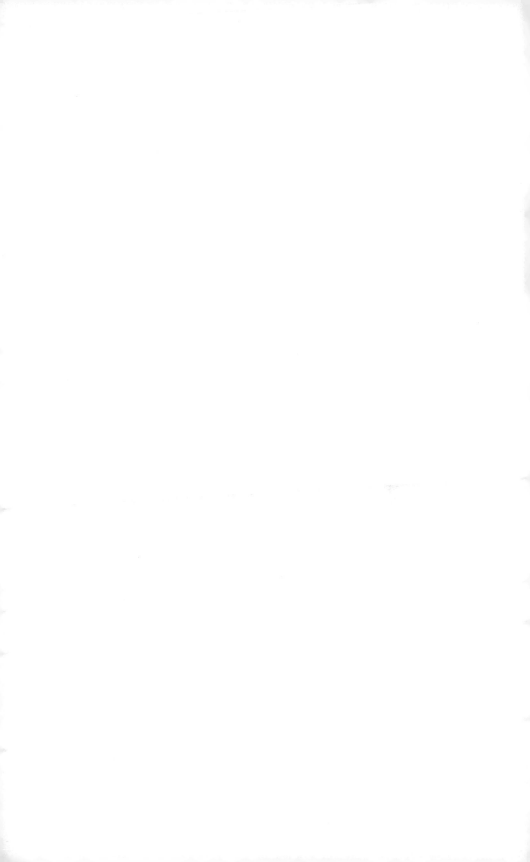

SUCCESS STORY:
Elizabeth Lovsin

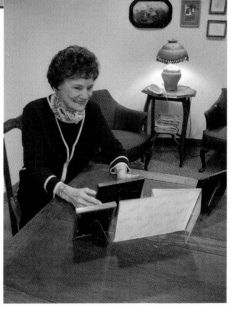

It's not unusual for people to feel a little nervous about their first visit to a new doctor, especially when the topic is a surgical procedure. But when Elizabeth first arrived at my office, she had reason to be more than a little nervous.

One sad day in May 1999, Elizabeth Lovsin's 48-year-old son failed to take the medications that kept his nearly lifelong battle with schizophrenia in check. In an uncharacteristic but catastrophic burst of violence, he shot and killed his beloved father and then turned the gun on his mother. Elizabeth was hit four times: in the wrist, the upper arm, the stomach, and the face. The shot to her face severed a slice from her tongue and shattered all but four of her lower teeth.

Widowed violently at 72, her ill son locked away from her in jail, her two daughters living out of state where frequent visiting was complicated because of her extensive physical rehabilitation requirements, Elizabeth became depressed and discouraged.

"I like to talk. I like to sing. I enjoy food," she says. These everyday pleasures had been taken from her, along with two of the people she loved most. Worse, as the months passed, "I couldn't imagine what was going to change any of it."

The temporary measure taken to replace the eleven shattered teeth in her lower jaw, wasn't helping. A temporary partial denture had been secured to her remaining lower teeth, but it wasn't very stable.

Elizabeth Lovsin:

I hesitated over the cost. But then, everyone told me I needed to do this for myself. They were right. I needed encouragement, and Dr. Babbush gave it to me. Just talking to him that first time lifted my spirits more than I can describe. You lose track of the fact that you have an artificial object in your mouth. God Bless Dr. Babbush. He reshaped my future.

"It would never stay in place," she says. "I had so many problems with eating that I lost a tremendous amount of weight. And I was very, very self-conscious about my speech. I'd been in speech therapy, but speaking was still just terrible."

At the rehab center where she worked through her other injuries, she was told she needed dental implants; a friend who worked in another dental office gave her my name. Her sense of desperation growing, she made an appointment.

"I was apprehensive," she says about her initial visit in November 1999. "I had no idea what a 'dental implant' even was."

The appointment addressed that particular void quickly. A retired teacher, Elizabeth underwent an immediate education about dental implant treatment in general and dental implant treatment for her. At the end of the appointment, she recalls, "Dr. Babbush told me, 'I think maybe we can help you. Maybe we can get you eating again, talking again, functioning again.' The critical thing was making sure there was enough bone left in my lower jaw to hold the implants."

A CT scan confirmed the bone was sufficient. After that, only one hurdle remained, and it was quickly overcome.

"I hesitated over the cost," she says. "But then everyone told me I needed to do this for myself. They were right."

In a patient with less realism, the psychological impact of Elizabeth's tragedy might have given a doctor pause. But Elizabeth Lovsin is nothing if not realistic. She knew implants could only replace her teeth, not anything else she'd lost. She also knew she had to start rebuilding her life somewhere, and regaining the ability to eat and talk, to laugh and sing was a very good place.

"I could talk to therapists until I was blue in the face," she says. "The fact was that I needed to do something with my mouth."

By the time her first implant appointment was over, Elizabeth says she experienced an emotion she hadn't felt since the shooting: hope.

"I had lost my husband. My son was in jail. I needed encouragement, and Dr. Babbush gave it to me," she says. "Just talking to him that first time lifted my spirits more than I can describe." When all her diagnostics were complete and the surgery was scheduled, she signed the consent form with an overwhelming sense of relief.

Two months after her initial implant appointment, Elizabeth checked into an outpatient surgery center. The four remaining root tips and teeth in her lower jaw were removed, and her jawbone was built up with platelet-rich plasma combined with bone-graft materials. Six implants were placed alongside four temporary implants. Interim teeth were placed on the four temporary implants at the end of the surgical procedure. The surgery and her recovery were uneventful. In August 2000, her case was finished when a clip-bar overdenture was delivered by the restorative dentist, whose dental hygienist had first referred her.

Dental implants took the pain and discomfort out of eating and speaking for Elizabeth. Though the injury to her tongue continues to cause some abnormal sensations within her mouth, she says she can barely tell the difference between her natural upper teeth and replacement lower teeth. "You lose track of the fact that you have an artificial object in your mouth."

There is, of course, still pain in her life. A year after the shootings, Elizabeth's son died in prison. Though she had been angry at first over his actions, her anger eventually gave way to her knowledge that the violence was the work of her son's illness, not his heart. Her words falter when she says that she was rarely allowed to see her son and never allowed to hug him, not once, after the shooting. As his victim, it was considered unsafe.

The falter is brief. Self-pity isn't in this former teacher's workbook.

"It could have been even worse," she says. "I could have died. I could have been left an invalid."

For Elizabeth, dental implants were the turning point.

"God bless Dr. Babbush," she says. "He reshaped my future."

5 *What Happens Below the Gums*

From June Goldberg's unusual vantage point, one thing stands out about the evolution of dental implant surgery in the last quarter-century: the number of people present in the operating room.

June is the happy recipient of two dental implants—one placed in early 1975 and the second placed nearly 27 years later, in late 2001 (Figure 5.1).

"The first time, the surgery was done in the hospital, and implants were still very experimental," June recalls.

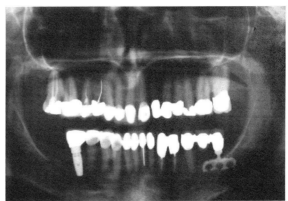

Figure 5.1 June Goldberg's panoramic x-ray shows the 26-year-old blade-vent implant that was placed in 1975 on the lower right. On the lower left, the endosteal implant placed in 2001 can be seen.

"Dr. Babbush was one of the few oral surgeons in America even carrying out these procedures.

"There we were in an operating room inside the hospital, and I remember the room being filled with people. Most of them were other dentists or residents training to learn how to do this new procedure. I remember waking up and saying, 'That didn't take long!' and there was a big laugh from the crowd."

73

By the time June fractured a molar in early 2001 and decided to replace the tooth with her second implant, implant surgery was a routine procedure performed more than half a million times a year in the United States alone. As a patient, June says she didn't notice any real difference in the surgery or recovery, but she did notice that the procedure seemed more ordinary.

"The second time around, the surgery took place in the office, and the only people there were the doctor and his assistants. It was pretty quiet."

Where Your Surgery is Performed

Most implant surgeries today are carried out like June's second one, in the private dental office or dental clinic of your clinician. These are "implant-friendly" settings where the equipment and personnel are dedicated to implant procedures. It is easy for doctors to perform surgery in these familiar settings where they work daily, and many patients feel more comfortable in the dental office than in a more hospital-like setting.

If your implant treatment plan is relatively straightforward and you have no complicating medical or other factors, chances are your dentist will recommend that your surgery take place in the office, where you will be attended by dental assistants rather than medical personnel such as operating room nurses. On the other hand, if your implant treatment plan is complex or you have pre-existing medical conditions, your doctor may recommend that your surgery be performed in an outpatient-surgery center or possibly in a hospital where you can be observed overnight following the procedure.

Situations that commonly prompt dentists to place implants in settings other than their own offices or clinics include the following:

If your surgical procedure will be lengthy or complex

A perfect example of a "complex" implant case is one in which bone is being harvested from the knee or hip and grafted into the jaw. In these cases, a general anesthetic is usually used, and in some instances another clinician, such as an orthopedic surgeon, may be involved to harvest the bone material. In this or any case that involves multiple procedures and/or multiple clinicians, many dentists prefer to work in a formal operating room.

If you have complicating medical conditions

High blood pressure, heart disease, respiratory disease, and a number of other chronic medical conditions can complicate dental implant treatment. Richard Miller, the Success Story who received implants after suffering a life-threatening heart infection, was treated in a hospital and observed overnight following his surgery as a precaution because of his potential for developing another heart infection and the resulting necessity for intravenous antibiotics. When a complicating medical condition is present, your dentist may consult with your physician about the best setting and the best type of anesthetic for your implant surgery. A recommendation or requirement that your procedure take place in a surgery center or hospital may result.

If you feel more comfortable in a hospital or surgical center

Any implant candidate who feels more comfortable in a hospital or hospital-like setting may elect this option after in-depth discussion with the surgeon.

Preparing for Surgery

Wherever your surgery takes place, you will be given a set of instructions to help prepare you for your implant surgery.

Blood thinners

If you are taking any kind of blood thinner—which may include aspirin, aspirin-based compounds, vitamin E, gingko biloba, ibuprofen, or prescription anticoagulants such as Coumadin—you will be instructed to stop taking these pills prior to surgery. By thinning the blood, these medicines increase the risk of excessive bleeding during and/or after any surgical procedure.

In the case of non-prescription drugs that have the effect of thinning your blood, you will probably be asked to stop ten days to two weeks before your surgery. In the case of prescription anticoagulants, your physician will be consulted, and you will be asked to stop taking your pills or lower your dosage from one to five days before surgery.

Patients who take prescription or non-prescription drugs for arthritis or other problems may substitute acetaminophen or Tylenol-based medications in the weeks leading up to surgery because these do not thin the blood.

Smoking

If you smoke, you will be advised to attempt to stop at least two weeks before your implant surgery. Smoking impairs your blood circulation, which is vital to prompt and complete post-operative healing. Studies have found that the constriction of blood circulation typical in smokers can be reversed or significantly reduced in a two-week period. Better blood supply means better healing and surer success. These benefits are greatly enhanced if you abstain for smoking for six to eight weeks following the surgery.

Food and liquids

If you are to receive anything other than a local anesthetic for your surgery (e.g., twilight or intravenous sedation or general anesthesia), you will be instructed to stop taking food or liquids many hours before the operation—usually the night before. That's because some patients experience nausea as a side effect of sedation or anesthesia. Vomiting undigested food while you are not fully alert can lead to a serious complication if the effluence is breathed (aspirated) into your lungs.

When the surgical appointment is in the afternoon, the doctor may modify this instruction to allow you to take some nourishment such as clear liquids very early in the day.

Antibiotics

Patients who are having a tooth removed in conjunction with their implant placement are typically placed on antibiotics three to five days before implant surgery. This precautionary measure is taken to reduce the chance that any active infection will be present at the implant site when surgery takes place. Even if no tooth is being removed, patients with pre-existing medical conditions that make them vulnerable to infection also will be placed on so-called "prophylactic" antibiotics. These typically include people with a history of rheumatic heart disease, an artificial heart valve, mitral valve prolapse with regurgitation, or any artificial joint replacement (e.g., hip, knee).

Corticosteroids

Patients who take corticosteroids for conditions such as advanced rheumatoid arthritis or certain dermatological disorders are in the opposite situation from patients taking blood thinners: they may need a *higher* dosage of medication than normal. The adrenal gland is suppressed when you take a therapeutic level of corticosteroids over a long period of time. Because the stress of anesthesia and a surgical procedure often suppresses the adrenal gland anyway, an extra dose on the day of surgery may be recommended to keep your adrenal gland functioning at its normal level.

The Day of Surgery

When you arrive for your surgical appointment, you will probably be asked if you followed all the pre-operative instructions you were given ahead of time. If you've forgotten to stop taking your daily aspirin or you absent-mindedly ate breakfast, it's important to 'fess up. The same is true if you're asked whether you have a cold or are running a fever. Your surgery will be cancelled if you are ill. Rescheduling your surgery will inconvenience you, your doctor, and the staff, but it is better than undergoing a procedure when proper precautions have not been taken.

You will probably be asked if you have made arrangements to be driven home as previously instructed once the procedure is finished. If your surgery is being performed under anything other than a local anesthetic of the sort you'd receive to have a tooth filled, you cannot safely drive. Sedation of any kind, even nitrous oxide—which may feel as if it dissipates the instant you stop receiving it—can continue to impair your ability to operate a motor vehicle safely.

Once the front office has verified all your preparations, you will be escorted to the operatory where your doctor will join you. Don't be surprised if he or she asks again about the preparations you took before coming to the appointment. "Better safe than sorry" is a common approach to pre-operative precautions; you're likely to be asked the same questions several times before the anesthetic is administered.

If you are receiving intravenous sedation or nitrous oxide, you will enter a "twilight" state once anesthesia is started and will probably be only vaguely aware of what takes place after that point. Before that moment, however, you will undergo these preparatory steps:

- A blood-pressure cuff will be placed on your arm
- Your body and clothing will be draped
- If you have long hair, a surgical cap may be used to cover it
- If you are receiving a local anesthetic, the area may be numbed topically with a gel
- If you are receiving IV sedation, a tourniquet will be placed on the arm that doesn't hold the blood-pressure cuff

If you will be sedated during the procedure, it is possible that one or more devices in addition to the blood-pressure cuff will be used to monitor how you're doing throughout the procedure. These may include blood pressure, continuous electrocardiogram (EKG), and/or pulse oximeter, which measures oxygen content in the blood and usually provides a pulse reading at the same time. All are safeguards that the doctor uses, just as you use a seatbelt when you ride in a car. They will usually be initiated before anesthesia is started.

Anesthetic

Local anesthesia is the most familiar form of anesthetic used for implant surgery. It is a site-specific medication that numbs the implant site so that you do not experience unpleasant or painful sensations during the surgical procedures.

Many implant patients opt to undergo their implant surgery under a combination of local anesthesia and some kind of "twilight" sedation. Twilight sedation is administered intravenously (via a needle placed in a vein) or via inhalation (through a mask placed over your nose). Though you may feel oblivious to what's going on around you, you can answer questions if asked, and you maintain all your reflexes.

When a general anesthetic is administered, the procedures are similar to the ones used for sedation, but the drug's effect is much more profound. You are "asleep" as opposed to being deeply dreamy. You cannot answer questions, and you lose your reflexes.

Whether "twilight" or complete, today's advanced forms of sedation and anesthesia take effect extremely quickly—within two or three minutes—and typically wear off rapidly.

Surgical Scenarios

The procedure described below applies to the placement of endosseous implants, which account for roughly 95 percent of all the dental implants placed today. If you are being treated with an alternative type of implant (i.e., subperiosteal, transosteal), the procedure will be different. Your doctor will be the best source of specific information for any alternative type of treatment planned for you.

There are two basic approaches to placing endosseous implants. In the "classic" approach, the implants are placed at one surgery, after which the tissues are allowed to heal for four to six months. At the end of this period, a second surgery is performed to "uncover" the buried implants and install a post called a healing abutment that brings the implant up through the gum tissue. This is known as "two-stage" treatment and is the approach pioneered by Brånemark in the 1960s. The second approach, which was introduced more than 20 years ago and has grown recently in popularity, eliminates the second-stage surgery. Implants are placed and immediately fitted with an abutment. Temporary replacement teeth may also be fitted the day of surgery.

Whether you're undergoing one-stage or two-stage implant treatment, the procedure for placing the implant itself is identical. An incision is made through the gum tissue, and the tissues are folded back to reveal the jaw structure underneath. What happens next depends upon the dental condition that already exists.

Implant insertion without the extraction of teeth

If the tooth or teeth being replaced by implants were lost prior to the implant surgery, and the extraction socket is healed, your bony tissue is ready for surgery. This is the most straightforward of implant cases. From a surgical standpoint, all that remains is determining whether you have enough bone to hold the implant(s). If the bone is sufficient, the implants are placed.

Extraction with immediate implant placement

If a tooth or teeth must be extracted because of decay, breakage, or compromise by gum disease, the tooth/teeth will be removed, but the placement of the implants will depend on whether infection is present. Reducing the chance of acute infection is why your dentist may have placed you on antibiotics a few days before the procedure. If s/he opens your gum tissue and finds no acute infection (e.g., pus) and enough bone to proceed, the implants are placed.

Extraction with delayed implant placement

If infection is present when your tooth is extracted, the site will be cleaned and the tissue closed without placing your implant. You will continue taking your antibiotics and return at a later date, usually in several weeks, after the infection is gone, for implant placement.

Extraction with staged implant placement

If there is no infection, but there is also not enough bone, additional bone material will be "grafted" into the implant site to build up what is already there. This bone-graft material can come from any one of several sources: the patient (chin, hip, knee); freeze-dried human bone; freeze-dried animal bone; or an artificial source such as hydroxyapatite. These materials are described in the next chapter.

The Surgical Procedure

Implants come in many sizes and in more than one shape. A single patient may receive implants of several different sizes because conditions may vary at each implant site in the same mouth. To prepare your jawbone for your implant(s), the dentist uses a sequence of precision surgical burs to drill a hole that precisely matches the implant selected for each site. In some cases, platelet-rich plasma fabricated from three-quarters of an ounce of your own blood—drawn immediately prior to the surgery and prepared to concentrate your platelets—is placed in the site to enhance healing.

Once the site is drilled to the proper depth, the implant is tapped or screwed into the hole until the implant is fully and firmly seated. Depending on whether you are undergoing two-stage or one-stage treatment, a healing screw or cap is threaded into the top of the implant, or an abutment is placed.

The doctor then sutures the gum tissue closed. Your implants are in place, and you are ready to begin healing. The matter of what you use for replacement teeth while healing is taking place and your final prosthesis is being crafted will be described fully in the next chapter (Figures 5.2A-F).

Figures 5.2A-F The sequence of the placement of an endosteal (in the bone) implant:

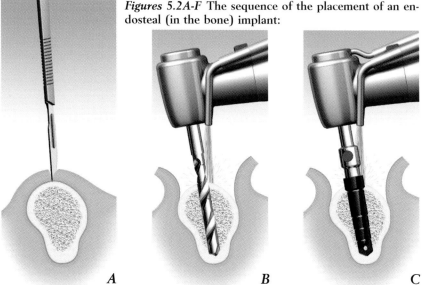

A   B   C

A) An incision is made in the gum with a scalpel.
B,C) A series of drills are used to prepare the site in the jawbone for placement of the implant.

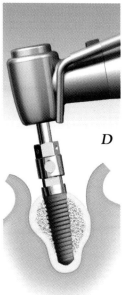

D

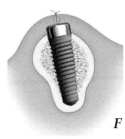

D) The implant is placed into the socket in the jawbone.
E) Once the implant is in the final position, the sealing screw is placed.

E

F) The gum tissue is replaced over the jawbone and implant, and a suture is placed. The implant is then allowed to heal before the gum tissue is reopened, and the crown is connected to the implant.

F

After the Surgery

Immediately following the surgery, you will continue resting in the dental chair or move into a designated recovery area until you feel alert and able to be driven home. You will leave the office with written and oral post-operative instructions that will include diet and hygiene guidelines, a prescription for medication to moderate any discomfort and possibly for antibiotics. You will also have an appointment to return for a check-up, usually within a week.

Food and drink

For the 24 hours following the surgery, you should avoid food or drink that is hot. Heat can cause or increase bleeding. Anything with sharp edges should be avoided as well. Chips, popcorn, crusty bread, and even salad greens can jab your fresh wound and cause irritation or bleeding. Food and liquids high in citric acid (e.g., oranges, grapefruit, and their juices) easily irritate the sensitized gastrointestinal tract. If you don't normally eat yogurt, now is not the time to start; it, too, can cause gastric problems. Ice cream and milkshakes are discouraged because they are rich and may cause nausea. Sorbet, Popsicles, or ice chips, on the other hand, are not a problem. And you should drink *lots* of fluids—carbonated sodas, apple juice, ice tea and, of course, water.

Antibiotics

If antibiotics have been prescribed to treat an active infection or to prevent one from developing, it is extremely important to take these pills as directed until all the pills are gone. It is ineffective and, in some cases, dangerous to take some of the pills, stop, then start taking them again.

Pain medication

The need for pain medication is highly individual. June Goldberg recalls experiencing no pain after either of her implant surgeries. "I was given a prescription, which I filled, but I threw the pills out without ever opening the bottle," she recalls.

Other patients manage mild discomfort with an over-the-counter painkiller such as Extra-Strength Tylenol, which does not contain any blood-thinning agents that might increase your bleeding. Patients who experience greater discomfort may take the painkillers that have been prescribed. Dentists typically take the better-safe-than-sorry approach and give all patients a prescription for pain medication, in case they fall into the last category.

Ice and rinsing

You will probably be asked to ice your jaw where your implants were placed because the cold both decreases the chances of bleeding and reduces swelling, which slows healing. An ice bag, ice pack, or unopened bag of frozen peas can be used. Just be sure you don't apply the frozen pack directly to your bare skin. It hurts! Wrap it in a lightweight towel first.

You will also begin rinsing your mouth well several times a day with lukewarm tap water mixed in equal parts with your choice of mouth rinse. Rinsing is done after every meal, when you wake up in the morning, and when you go to bed at night, and it continues until your first post-operative appointment with your doctor. Proper rinsing can speed healing.

Cleaning

You should not try to clean your surgical sites with anything but the lukewarm rinses, but you should continue brushing the remaining teeth in your mouth. Just take care to avoid irritating the site of your surgery. A Q-tip dipped into the water-mouthwash solution you are using for rinsing allows you to clean closer to the site itself.

The Healing Period

Healing after implant surgery takes place in two phases. The duration and intensity of these periods varies with the complexity and magnitude of your surgery, any pre-existing medical conditions you might have, and any medications you take on a daily basis. The following schedule applies to most patients.

Phase One: 3-5 days

The first phase typically lasts three to five days and is the most uncomfortable stage. Whatever tenderness, sensitivity, swelling, and/or bruising you experience will be greatest during this interval. You may feel swelling and pain in your ears or under the lower jaw, on the side of your head, under your eyes, or along the side of your nose. The surgical site in your mouth may appear white. This is normal. It is your mouth's equivalent of the red scab that forms on your skin when you scrape or cut yourself.

You may also experience some bloody oozing for up to 48 hours after your surgery. If the bleeding is heavy, you can treat it by rinsing your mouth several times with warm water, using gauze to gently clean the area, and then biting firmly down on a half-inch wad of gauze placed over the bleeding area. To decrease bleeding, you will need to maintain pressure for 30 minutes without removing the gauze.

Even if you feel well the day after surgery, it is wise to take it easy for up to five days—especially during the first two days following your procedure. Avoid social engagements and extended telephone calls that require you to overwork your jaw with speech. Abstain from sports activities, including workouts. The whole purpose of fitness activities is to increase your blood pressure and blood supply. This is counterproductive when you are recovering from any surgical procedure, including implant placement. Increasing your pulse rate can delay healing, cause

When to Call Your Doctor

If you experience any of the following post-operative complications, a telephone call to your doctor is warranted.

- *Excessive bleeding (copious bleeding that cannot be controlled by rinsing and/or applying pressure with gauze to the site)*
- *Excessive swelling (swelling that distorts facial features)*
- *Pain that is not controlled by your prescription medication*
- *Nausea/vomiting*
- *Signs of allergic reaction (e.g., rash or itching associated with antibiotics or other medications)*

bleeding, or increase/cause throbbing and/or pain at the site(s) of your surgery.

Phase Two: 10-14 days

After these first few days, the second stage of healing begins. This will last roughly 10 to 14 days, during which time any unpleasant post-surgical side effects you felt immediately after the surgery will subside gradually and eventually disappear. During this period, you can return to your normal diet as it becomes comfortable to you. Patients who receive temporary teeth at the same time implants are placed may remain on a modified diet for somewhat longer. If you normally take prescription anticoagulants, you will resume taking them as directed by your doctor.

Following Up

Your doctor will want to see you approximately a week after your surgery to check on your post-operative progress. S/he will look at the healing and color of your tissues, make sure your sutures are holding, and confirm that there's no unusual swelling or bleeding. Your antibiotic regime will be reviewed, and the use of blood thinners will be re-evaluated in light of your overall medical condition. A program of oral hygiene and maintenance for the months until your implants are restored will be established. This appointment is typically brief.

In the weeks and months that follow, your doctor may ask you to return to the office regularly so s/he can continue to monitor your healing process and give you a chance to ask questions. These very short appointments are the equivalent of a routine visit to your dentist and are just as important. They are preventative, helping to assure smooth and complete healing before you move into the next phase: uncovering your implants and receiving your final new teeth.

David Hanbury

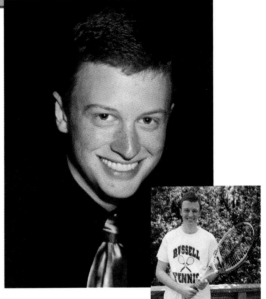

Implants improve the lives of people of all ages, as David's story demonstrates. But young as he is, he is not unique. I see many young adults in my practice.

The Tooth Fairy never came to collect David Hanbury's baby teeth. But it wasn't the Tooth Fairy's fault.

Today a normal, healthy 16-year-old from Ashland, Kentucky, David was about six years old when he and his parents learned something was amiss. The revelation came during a routine dental appointment with the family's dentist, when an x-ray revealed that David lacked the permanent tooth buds that most children develop as preschoolers. This condition is known as anodontia.

Anodontia is a genetic disorder. Indeed one of David's brothers also was missing some of his permanent teeth, and one cousin had never developed any. As David's friends and classmates began losing their teeth, David's parents tried to help their son cope with his condition as well as possible. They arranged for the Tooth Fairy to leave money for David whenever one of his brothers lost a tooth. On a more practical note, they began having dentures made for David when he was in the fifth grade.

Dentures were necessary because David's baby teeth were "very, very tiny," his mother recalls. "Also, they had worn down throughout the years. So they didn't look right." Four molars and one of the upper front teeth finally did develop, but these came in behind the baby teeth, instead of displacing them.

The dentures made for David fit over his upper teeth and allowed the boy to eat and speak fairly well. (His lip concealed his lower teeth well enough that he was able to forego wearing dentures over them.) But David had a series of problems with the upper denture. The framework broke a couple of times, and individual teeth also broke off from the plate. As David's mouth grew, further adjustments were necessary to accommodate the growth.

"Finally they came up with a metal-lined overdenture that wouldn't break," David recalls. But he says, "My second home seemed to be the dentist's office."

Although most people probably didn't notice he was wearing dentures, David felt they looked artificial. This is a normal reaction among adolescents, who are particularly prone to embarrassment and uncertain self-esteem. So when David learned about dental implants, he was immediately interested. "I knew going in that this was going to be something I would invest a lot of time in. But I was so tired of dentures I was ready to do it."

> **David Hanbury:**
> *The difference in the way they look is huge. They look amazingly better. Despite all the time that the treatment required. I never once questioned my decision that implants were the right thing. I never looked back.*

Faced with the prospect of major dental implant surgery, David's parents consulted a close family friend who was an oral surgeon.

"He'd been following David's case all along, and he knew Dr. Babbush and had read his articles," David's mother says. "Our friend would have done the case if it had just involved one or two implants. But because David needed such extensive work, we decided to go to Dr. Babbush in Cleveland, even though it was five hours away."

In Cleveland, David was examined, and a complete set of x-rays and a CT scan were taken. A sophisticated computer program and consultation with the restorative dentist also helped to determine the best way to restore David's mouth. Presented with this plan, David and his parents agreed to proceed with treatment.

On June 7, 2002, the family again made the five-hour drive from Ashland to Cleveland, and David checked into the surgi-center. Because of the scope of the work to be done, he was given general anesthesia. In the course of a nine-hour surgery, all 19 of his baby teeth were extracted, along with the one permanent central incisor, which was severely misaligned. These were replaced with 18 dental implants. Because David's jaw-bone had shrunk due to the absence of permanent teeth, some bone grafting also was done. Platelet-rich plasma was used to improve the bone quality and quantity, as well as to speed the healing process. Upper and lower temporary prostheses were then anchored to the one permanent molar that David remained in each of the four quadrants of David's mouth and to some of the implants. A few days later, David returned home with func-tional temporary teeth.

The year that followed further tested David's impatience with dental offices. He and his parents had to make the ten-hour round trip for weekly and then biweekly check-ups at first, and a few unexpected events also brought him back to Cleve-land for additional work. When he disregarded the instructions he'd been given to avoid solid food, his temporary restoration cracked at one point and had to be replaced.

Second-stage surgery to uncover the implants was carried out in November of 2002. The temporary teeth were adjusted and replaced in David's mouth at that time. At no point in his treatment did he have to function without teeth. In February of 2003, David returned to the restorative dentist, and impressions were taken in order to fabricate his permanent teeth. He received these by summer 2003.

"The difference in the way they look is huge," David says. "They look amazingly better." Any self-consciousness he once felt about his teeth has rapidly evaporated. Despite all the time that the treatment required, David says he never once questioned his decision that implants were the right thing for him. "I had made up my mind completely, and I've never looked back," he says.

6 When You Need More Than Implants

Experienced gardeners know that if you plant a strong and healthy shrub where it will get the perfect amount of light and water, it still may suffer if the ground lacks certain key components. A good foundation is essential.

Implants are no different.

The most skillful implant doctor can place the best-designed implant in a patient who is meticulous about oral hygiene, and things may still go badly if some basic elements are missing. The implant site must have sufficient:

- Quality and quantity of bone
- Gum tissue
- Anatomical structure

Unfortunately, tooth decay and gum disease tend to degrade these conditions, as does tooth loss, since the absence of a tooth changes the anatomy at the site. Fortunately for today's patients, techniques for solving such problems have developed.

This chapter describes the most common procedures performed when the foundation for dental implants needs to be improved.

Bone Grafting

Bone grafting is by far the most common supplementary procedure in implant dentistry, performed in close to 90 percent of all patients. If a patient doesn't have enough bone to ensure that his or her implants will be successful, the doctor in the vast majority of cases can create new bone. This is possible because of the human body's remarkable ability to regenerate bone. Whereas other parts of the body heal by growing scar tissue, bone that is formed after an injury or disease eventually cannot be distinguished from the original tissue. It is literally as good as new.

Bone grafting triggers this act of magic. Dentists typically use one of four types of bone-graft materials: autografts, allografts, alloplasts, and/or xenografts.

Autografts

When bone is taken from one part of the body to be used in another part of the same person's body, this is known as an autograft. Common harvest sites include the chin, the hip, the knee, and the part of the jaw behind the molars (Figure 6.1). The void left where bone has been taken is then usually repaired with one of the alloplast or xenograft materials discussed below.

The harvesting of autograft (or "autogenous") bone may require a separate surgery, or it may take place during the

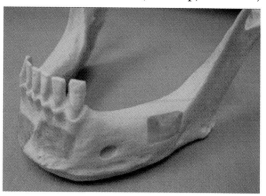

Figure 6.1 A model of the lower jaw demonstrates the areas from which autograft bone can be harvested (orange squares). The harvested bone can then be used for grafting procedures inside the mouth.

same operation in which the implants are placed. When the bone is being taken from the patient's chin or mouth, the operation typically is performed in the doctor's office, although more complex cases may dictate the use of an outpatient surgery center. If a larger amount of bone is required, the doctor may have to obtain the material from the hip or knee. A surgery center or hospital (where an overnight stay might be necessary) almost always is the setting for such operations, and the doctor should have had special training in bone-graft harvesting. Most oral surgeons receive such training. Sometimes orthopedic surgeons also are involved in harvesting bone from the hip or knee.

Autografts offer two principal benefits. The patient runs no risk of disease infection when the bone comes from his or her own body. Secondly, because it's fresh, autogenous bone contains live cells that will promote the healing process.

The obvious drawback to using autogenous bone is that the patient must be operated on in two places. This increases

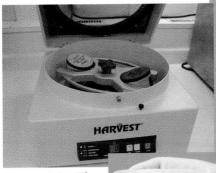

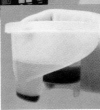

Figure 6.9A The Harvest Technology machine, which fabricates platelet concentrate.

Figure 6.9B The platelet button (concentrate) can be seen at the bottom of the processing container.

Platelet Rich Plasma

The major components of normal blood are plasma, red cells, white cells, and platelets. Platelets are tiny cells that play an important role in helping blood to form a clot at a wound site. They also contain reservoirs of growth factors that stimulate the body's natural healing process.

Methods developed decades ago can increase the concentration of these platelets, producing so-called platelet-rich plasma (PRP). Placing this material in the surgical wound results in reduced bleeding, decreased inflammation and swelling, improved wound closure, accelerated bone regeneration, and faster overall healing time. Platelet-rich plasma has become an increasingly important ingredient in bone- and gum-grafting operations, as well as other types of surgical reconstruction.

Today's technology makes it possible for the doctor to produce platelet-rich plasma from just a small amount of normal blood. Right before surgery, less than an ounce of blood is drawn from the patient. (In comparison, donors in blood-collection drives typically give 16 ounces of blood.) The patient's blood is immediately placed into a special centrifuge and spun at very high speed for 14 minutes. This separates the platelets from the red and white blood cells. By adjusting the amount of plasma in which the platelets are suspended, the doctor can concentrate the platelets to up to ten times the normal value (more than two million platelets per microliter, versus about 200,000 in ordinary blood). The concentrate is then applied as a gel to the areas being grafted. Nature takes care of the rest (Figures 6.9A,B).

the risk of post-operative discomfort and other complications from the surgery.

Allografts

When a doctor takes tissue from one person and transfers it to someone else, that's an allograft. Bone allografts usually are harvested from cadavers under sterile operating conditions, then immediately freeze-dried. Occasionally, a living person may donate bone.

In the past, allograft bone posed some risk of passing on a disease from the donor to the recipient. However, in recent years, certified tissue banks have developed stringent procedures for checking upon each donor's health history, as well as examining the bone for disease organisms. The tissue banks have also learned how to process the freeze-dried bone in ways that make it virtually impossible for any undetected disease organisms such as HIV (human immunodeficiency virus) or hepatitis to survive and/or be transferred to another person. Typically, the bone is immersed in graded alcohols and acids, freeze-dried (usually to -70C), and tested for pathogens again. This process is so rigorous that it has even been shown to kill HIV virus that was deliberately introduced into the bone by researchers.

Implant doctors can purchase freeze-dried allograft bone in a number of different forms. It may take the form of small granules resembling coarse salt or sand. It is also available in pieces that mimic the structure being augmented (Figures 6.2A,B).

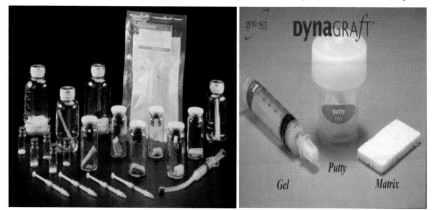

Figures 6.2A,B Various forms of allograft materials for bone grafting.

Allograft bone has the advantage of requiring no second surgery from the implant patient. While it contains fewer elements to stimulate growth than fresh living bone, research has demonstrated that some growth factors survive.

Alloplasts

This category includes ceramic materials that originate in substances such as South Sea coral. Such materials closely resemble the bone- mineral material contained in the human body. Always inert, alloplastic substances pose no threat of disease transmission. They also contain no growth factors, so this material

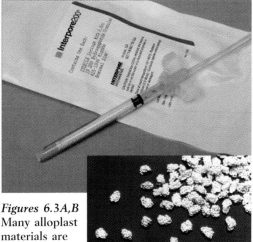

Figures 6.3A,B Many alloplast materials are delivered with a syringe-type apparatus and are granular in appearance.

cannot itself generate the development of new bone. Instead it serves as a bridge or "scaffold' into which surrounding bone can grow (Figures 6.3A,B).

Xenografts

Bone obtained from one species and transferred to another is called a xenograft. Most often the source is cattle. To mitigate concerns about transmitting bovine spongiform encephalopathy (better known as Mad Cow disease) and other cattle-borne disease, researchers have developed a process that eliminates any such threat. As with allografts and alloplasts, using xenografts spares the graft recipient the need for two surgical sites. Furthermore, even though the bone comes from an ani-

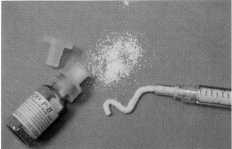

Figure 6.4 Xenograft material is available in a granular, as well gelatinous, form.

mal, studies have indicated that it not only serves as a scaffold for new bone growth but also contains elements that stimulate such growth (Figure 6.4).

All four categories of bone-grafting materials are commonly used in implant grafting procedures, either alone or in combination. The doctor usually will determine the best option for each case. However, any patient who has a strong preference for or against any particular type of graft material should air such concerns with the doctor.

The Timing of Bone Grafts

Bone can be built up either in preparation for implant placement or simultaneously with it. Conditions at the site usually dictate which approach will be necessary.

It has become common, for example, for doctors to place implants at the same time that they extract unsalvageable teeth. Because the shape of the extraction site almost never exactly matches the shape of the implant, some kind of a gap almost always exists and can be filled with bone-grafting material on the spot. Disease-induced bone loss or periodontitis at the extraction site may also increase the need for grafting. In cases where there's not enough bone at a site to support even the shortest or narrowest of implants, the doctor may need to place graft material and allow it to heal. Usually four to six months must pass before the graft is strong enough to allow for implant placement.

The floor of the sinuses in the upper jaw is an area where such two-stage grafting is common because, when teeth are lost from the sides of the upper jaw, the bone tends to thin dramatically, sometimes becoming thin as an eggshell. Such bone is far too thin to hold any implant in place. When this happens, the doctor can create an opening on the side of the sinus cavity, then insert bone-graft material in a quantity sufficient to accommodate implants later. Typically, this procedure involves only a small amount of additional discomfort, compared to standard implant placement. The incision required, as well as the anesthetic and post-operative medication, are the same. When enough

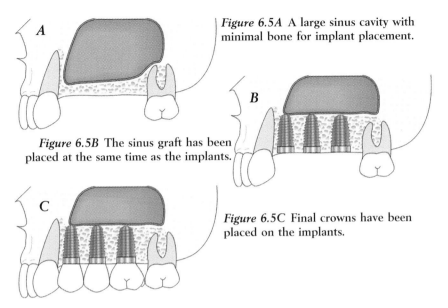

Figure 6.5A A large sinus cavity with minimal bone for implant placement.

Figure 6.5B The sinus graft has been placed at the same time as the implants.

Figure 6.5C Final crowns have been placed on the implants.

bone exists to allow for placement of implants, but the quantity isn't sufficient to ensure their success, sinus grafting can be done at the same time that the implants are placed (Figures 6.5A-C).

Soft-Tissue Grafting

As people age, it's common for their gum tissue to shrink. That's where the expression "long in the tooth" comes from. In fact, teeth don't grow longer, but they can appear to do so as the gum tissue recedes. Trauma, the presence of plaque, an overly hard toothbrush, inappropriate brushing techniques, and other oral factors all can take their toll on the soft tissue in the mouth.

For anyone having dental implants placed, the presence of good-quality gum tissue is important for several reasons. For one

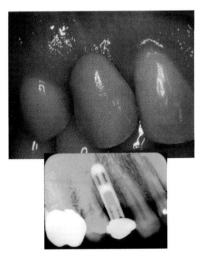

Figures 6.6A,B This photograph and x-ray show a single implant that has been in this patient's upper jaw for 14 years. Note the healthy gum tissue and natural appearance.

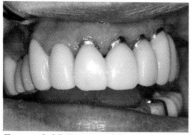

Figure 6.6C Poor oral hygiene often causes the gum tissue to recede around the implant.

thing, gum tissue that fits snugly around the implants acts as a barrier; it's the body's first line of defense against the bacteria that can cause periodontal disease and threaten the submerged implant. Secondly, healthy looking gum tissue is an important component of an attractive smile. Figures 6.6A-C illustrate the difference that the absence or presence of such tissue can make.

Between a quarter and a third of all dental implant patients require some form of soft-tissue grafting. As with bone, the skin required for soft-tissue grafts may be obtained from a second site in the patient. The palate and the inner part of the cheek are common traditional harvest sites. In recent years, more and more doctors have begun using freeze-dried donated skin to expand the amount of gum tissue available. Like freeze-dried bone, skin allografts nowadays undergo a complex screening and tissue-processing technique that has essentially eliminated any chance of disease transmission.

Regardless of the source of the graft material, the concept behind most soft-tissue grafting is simple. At the location where the additional gum tissue is needed, the doctor makes an incision. Then, like a seamstress enlarging a piece of clothing, s/he sews in a piece of graft material that has been cut to the proper shape. This may be done at the same time implants are placed or it may come later.

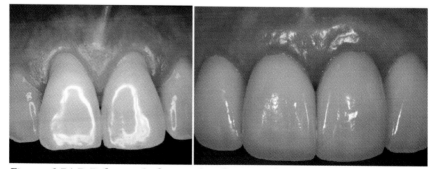

Figures 6.7A,B Before and after results of a gingival (gum) graft.

Recovery occurs in stages. Tenderness, swelling, and discomfort are greatest during the first three to five days. Over the next 10 to 12 days, these symptoms dissipate substantially. Within two to three months, the grafted area should look indistinguishable from the natural tissue. As with bone grafting, the success rate for soft-tissue grafting procedures is high; the use of platelet-rich plasma can increase it even more (Figures 6.7A,B).

Nerve Repositioning

Just as the loss of teeth from the upper jaw can decrease the space between the sinus and the gum surface, something similar happens in the lower jaw. When teeth are lost and the jawbone shrinks downward along with the gum surface, which gets closer and closer to the major nerve that enters the mouth at the back part of the jaw and runs under the molars. If the nerve gets close enough to the gum surface, any amount of pressure can

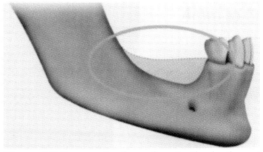

Figure 6.8 Progressive bone loss in the back part of a lower jaw has occurred in the wake of tooth extraction. The opening for the exit of the lower jaw nerve can be seen.

hurt so much that many patients with this condition can no longer tolerate wearing dentures (Figure 6.8).

Implants placed in a severely deteriorated lower jawbone are apt to hit the nerve—causing more pain and damage. One alternative in such cases is to build up the bone with a graft, making the jaw thick enough to hold the implants above the underlying nerve. However, the blocks of bone typically required for such cases must be taken from the hip, the chin, or the back portion of the lower jaw.

Nerve repositioning provides a way to avoid undergoing a block bone graft. In this operation, the doctor makes an incision in the gum, turns the tissue back, and creates a small window in the outside of the jawbone. Using special instruments, s/he gently grasps the nerve, and moves it to the side while implants are placed in the normal fashion. The nerve is then manipulated back into position—next to the newly placed implants but un-damaged by them.

Nerve-repositioning has a significant drawback. Some amount of nerve damage and loss of sensation is likely to follow this surgery. Since the nerve involved does not control any muscles, no paralysis nor any kind of facial disfigurement occurs. Instead the effect of any nerve damage is sensory. Most patients who experience some loss of feeling compare it to having a long-acting local anesthetic—one that affects the lip, chin, tongue, floor of the mouth, and/or gum tissue. When this operation is performed by an expert surgeon, the majority of patients find that the numbness subsides in the weeks and months after the procedure, with the area eventually returning to normal. Even when a small amount of numbness remains, however, it may represent a satisfying tradeoff, as the next Success Story illustrates.

Martha Schaffran

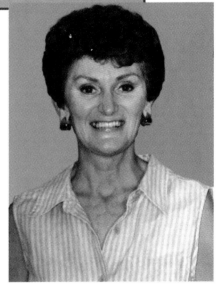

Some supplementary procedures have become routine in implant dentistry. Martha's was a little more unusual.

"When I was young, my parents didn't have the money for good dental care," Martha Schaffran says. When the Ohio resident developed cavities as a teenager, she recalls that the family dentist's solution was simple, if primitive: yank out any tooth that was causing problems. Soon, "I had three missing on one side and two on the other—which meant that I didn't have anything to chew on in the back," she says.

A partial denture solved that problem when Martha was in her 30s. "It was fine for a while," she says. "But then the partial started to hurt. I didn't realize that the reason was that the bone was getting thin. No one had ever told me that." By the time she reached her 40s, she was fitted with a new partial, but her relief from the chronic discomfort was short-lived. She soon felt as if her gums harbored shards of glass. "Wearing the partial was painful even if I wasn't chewing anything."

The pain drove her to abandon the partial denture and mash her food exclusively with the teeth in the front of her mouth. Over time, this unnatural motion damaged her incisors. Eventually, Martha had to have several of these front teeth extracted. Another denture, one cemented into place, served as a replacement for them.

Still, Martha says, she realized she needed teeth in the back of her mouth and relief from the pain there. Desperate for advice, she turned to the dental school at Case Western Reserve University, where I met with her. I advised her that the ridge of her jawbone had grown so thin she could never again expect it to support a conventional bridge. Indeed the bone was so thin that even yawning too hard might break her jaw. Implants offered her the only hope of a return to a normal life.

I advised her that in order to place two implants on each side, the nerve located within each side of her lower jaw would have to be temporarily moved. Grafting with particles of freeze-dried bone would also be necessary, and the use of platelet-rich plasma would increase the chances that the entire complex would heal well.

When Martha listened to a description of the numbness that might result from the nerve repositioning, it was a little like "being told that you have cancer," she recalls. "It scared me out of my mind!" She talked to other family members, and the majority of them warned her against proceeding. "I pictured myself looking like a stroke victim afterwards, where you're drooling and everything."

"I remember not being able to make a decision about whether I was going to be brave enough to do that. I wasn't so much afraid of the pain as I was of all these side effects." Still, she

Martha Schaffran:

I have no pain at all when I chew. It's been like a miracle. I can't even believe that I'm able to have these teeth in the back. I am adamant that I made the right choice. You think about the things that people spend money on. Cars for example. But they rust! I'm 55 now and I hope to have a good number of additional years. I just feel fortunate that I found the treatment when I did.

decided to return with her husband to help her evaluate all the complex information. "It seemed like the second time I wasn't as scared, and I kind of absorbed everything better." With her husband's encouragement, she decided to proceed with the surgery.

Martha says in the first week that followed the nerve repositioning, much of her mouth continued to feel anesthetized. After a week or so, her mouth began to feel tingly, a sign of improvement that gradually continued over the months that followed.

Fourteen months after receiving her final prosthesis, Martha judged that more than 90 percent of the sensation had returned to her mouth. "Around my chin it's still not quite the way it used to be in an area about the size of a dime, but it's nothing that I can't live with," she stated. "And I have no pain at all when I chew. It's like a miracle! I just can't even believe that I'm able to have these teeth in the back."

Because of the gravity of Martha's situation, her treatment took almost a year and a half to complete, including several months of living with the numbness and tingling. Yet she is adamant that she made the right choice. "Absolutely. You think about the things that people spend money on. Cars, for example. But they rust. I'm 55 now and I hopefully have a good number of additional years. I just feel very fortunate that I found the treatment I did."

7 What Happens Above the Gums

When June Goldberg received her first implant in 1975, implant treatment consisted of two stages: implant surgery followed by restoration after a very short healing period. By the late 1970s and early 1980s, the standard had changed. Based on Brånemark's landmark research, implant treatment evolved into a three-part process:

1. Initial surgery to place the implants, followed by a healing period with the implant buried below the gum

2. Second surgery to uncover the implants and fit them with the abutment posts that connect the new teeth above the gums with the implants below

3. The fabrication and fitting of the teeth or "final restoration"

The Brånemark approach remains the dominant one, but implant dentistry is a dynamic field. New techniques and methods continue to emerge. As a result, both the events following implant surgery and the teeth that patients use in the interim between surgery and final restoration have become far more variable.

This chapter will describe the three steps that the majority of dental implant patients continue to take on the road to new implant-supported teeth, the shorter sequence that selected patients may follow, and the temporary restorations available with both.

Teeth While You Heal

One of the foremost questions on the mind of any prospective dental implant patient is: What do I use for teeth immediately after my implants are placed but before my final new teeth are

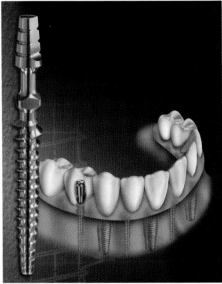

completed? No single answer applies to every patient. For some, interim teeth will be anchored by immediate provisional implants, one of the recent innovations in implant dentistry. Better known simply as IPIs, these implants address the question of interim teeth in an entirely new way. They are temporary miniature implants that are placed alongside the permanent implants during surgery and later removed.

Figure 7.1 The Immediate Provisional Implant (IPI) on the left and a diagram of its use in conjunction with regular implants.

They serve only one purpose: to secure a temporary, stable, functional restoration during the months when the implant sites are healing (Figure 7.1).

In some cases, a patient's existing denture can be hollowed out, modified, and cemented to the IPIs for the duration of the healing period. If you are one of these pa-

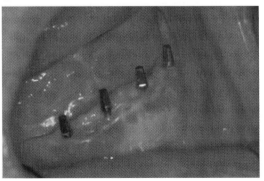

Figure 7.2 The healed lower jaw gum tissue with the temporary miniature implants in place.

tients, you may be able to wear teeth home on the day of surgery (Figures 7.2, 7.3).

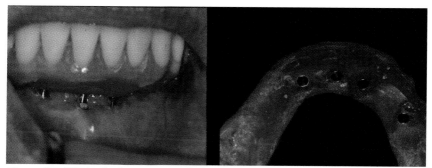

Figure 7.3 IPIs in the lower jaw with the little caps in the modified lower denture.

In other cases, a new "provisional" or temporary denture or bridge may be fabricated before your surgery by your dentist in conjunction with the dental laboratory to fit over the temporary implants. This option, too, may allow you to leave the surgical appointment with functioning teeth.

Even without IPIs, if you were wearing a full or partial denture before implant surgery, your doctor may be able to modify it to sit on your gums in such a way that no pressure is exerted on the implants beneath the surface. Premature pressure on healing implants can lead to potential complications and/or failure and is actively avoided. When dentures are modified to avoid such pressure, the patient typically is allowed to wear them after the first post-operative follow-up visit to the doctor. Modification and continued use of dentures in this way can reduce both the inconvenience and the expense of implant treatment.

If you are not a denture wearer at the time of your surgery, you and your dentist will consult and choose among a number of options for your provisional period:

Immediate restoration

When an implant is planned in the front of your mouth where teeth are highly visible, your dentist may place the implants and secure temporary crowns to them before you leave your surgical appointment. This is most commonly done when a tooth or teeth are being replaced individually (Figures 7.4A-D). When multiple teeth are being replaced, it is often more efficient to secure a partial or full denture with IPIs, as already described, or to your own natural teeth. Recently, alternatives such as Teeth in a Day™ and Brånemark-Novum™ have also emerged. These are techniques or systems that allow selected patients to leave the initial implant surgery with provisional and possibly even final restorations.

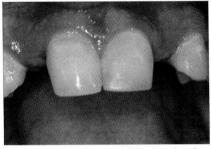 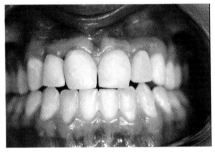

Figure 7.4A This patient failed to develop both lateral incisors in the upper jaw.

Figure 7.4B Two implants have been inserted and temporary crowns placed on the implants on the same day.

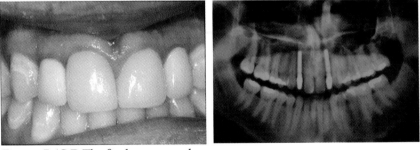

Figures 7.4C,D The final crowns and x-rays.

Removable prosthesis without IPI

A flipper or partial denture that looks much the same as the IPI-supported provisional denture but sits on the gums instead of attaching to the temporary implants may be a choice. These appliances can be more economical approach than using IPIs for the provisional stage. Like an existing denture that has been modified, a flipper or partial denture must be designed to prevent premature pressure on the implants.

No temporary restoration

If you have an implant placed in the back of the mouth where it is not visible, the appearance of the teeth may not be as important as it is in the front. If you do not have an existing prosthesis such as a partial denture or flipper to fill the void, you may decide simply to live with a gap while the underlying implant is healing. This is an economical approach to the provisional period that many patients find perfectly acceptable.

Second-Stage Surgery

Two-stage treatment requiring a second surgical procedure after the implants have fused with the bone remains the norm in implant treatment in this country. With this concept, a second surgery is performed after the gum tissue has healed and bone has grown onto the implant surface and become incorporated into the jaw itself. During this surgery, the gum tissue over the submerged implant is uncovered, and a small metal post is threaded into the implant. This may be a temporary healing abutment that will be replaced later or the final abutment that will anchor the ultimate restoration. In either case, this post serves as the connection between the implant below the gum and the restoration above it.

The timing of second-stage surgery is determined by the procedures that have preceded it.

In straightforward cases in which the implant was submerged beneath the gum, the gum tissue was sutured over it, and no additional surgical procedures were performed, second-stage surgery typically comes three to four months after the initial procedure. On the other hand, if the sinuses were grafted, a nerve was moved, or the jawbone was built up in conjunction with implant placement, the period between the first and second surgeries may extend for up to six months to allow the necessary healing for these additional procedures.

In cases where plenty of bone is available and an implant is placed in the less-visible back of the mouth, a healing abutment is sometimes placed into the implant at the same time the im-

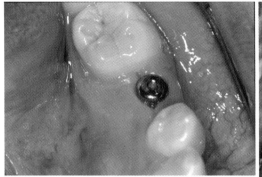

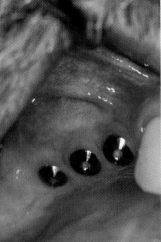

Figure 7.5A In this case, the healing abutment was placed at the time the implant was placed. Therefore, no second surgery was required.

plant is placed into the bone. This approach is called "one-stage" implant treatment because it eliminates the

Figure 7.5B One-stage placement shown for multiple implants.

need for the second surgery to expose the implants and place the abutments (Figures 7.5A,B). Patients who undergo one-stage implant treatment proceed directly to the restorative phase once their implants have healed. Otherwise, second-stage surgery is followed by a relatively short period during which the gums heal before the final, restorative phase of treatment—sometimes called the third stage of dental implant treatment—begins.

Second-stage surgery preparations

Pre-surgical preparations for your second-stage implant surgery will be similar but probably much less stringent than the ones that preceded your first surgery.

If you are taking blood thinners, you will be asked to discontinue them, whether they are prescription medications or a preventative aspirin-a-day. If you have a medical condition that requires prophylactic antibiotic treatment, you will be placed on it.

Except in rare cases when medical or other conditions require that you be treated in a surgical center, second-stage surgery usually will take place in your doctor's office. The vast majority of these surgeries are performed under local anesthetic without sedation so you probably will be given no special pre-treatment dietary instructions. Patients who do receive intravenous or twilight sedation or a general anesthetic will follow the same pre-operative protocols regarding food and liquids that were prescribed before their implant surgery.

If you have been wearing a cemented-in provisional restoration during the healing period, this restoration will have to be adapted again to accommodate the abutment placed at your second-stage surgery. If you are being treated by an implant team, it is possible that on the day of your second-stage surgery, you will first visit your restorative dentist for removal of your crown, bridge, or other temporary fixed teeth. You will then travel to your implant surgeon for your second-stage procedure, returning immediately afterwards to your restorative dentist/prosthodontist, who will modify your provisional appliance once again. The provisional is replaced over your abutments and secured.

Second-stage surgical procedure

When only one or some implants are involved, second-stage surgery is typically carried out with a simple application of local anesthetic to numb the gum tissue at the surgical site. If IPIs were placed at the first surgery, they will be removed at this time. The tissue is opened to expose the buried implant. This tissue often heals on its own without suturing. In some cases, one or more small, self-dissolving stitches may be necessary to bring the gum tissue back together.

Once the implant is exposed, the healing screw that was placed into its top at the time of initial surgery is removed. The implant is inspected to make sure it is solidly fused with the bone, and the surrounding gums are checked for health and vitality. The healing screw is replaced by either a healing abutment or the final abutment, depending on the circumstances (Figures 7.6, 7.7A). If the final

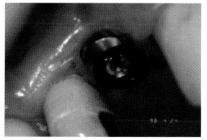

Figure 7.6 The healing abutment, once placed into the implant, extends up through the gum tissue.

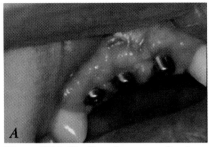

Figure 7.7A Healing abutments for three implants.

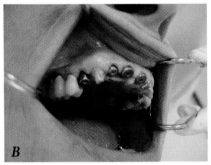

Figures 7.7B-C In this case, immediate temporary teeth were fabricated and placed the same day that the healing abutments were connected.

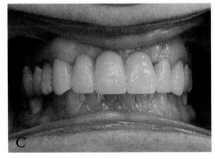

abutment is placed, it may be possible for a temporary crown or bridge to be fitted directly to the implants on that day (Figures 7.7B,C).

In any event, a period of time must follow the uncovering of the implant and placement of the abutment to allow the gums to fully heal and adapt before the impressions are taken for the final restoration, usually two to four weeks later.

Second-stage surgical recovery

Just as the preparations for second-stage surgery were much simplified, the aftermath typically is a great deal milder. Bleeding, swelling, pain, and other post-operative effects are likely to be minimal or non-existent. When one or a few implant sites are reopened, an over-the-counter medication such as Extra-Strength Tylenol, if anything, is typically all that's required for discomfort. Icing is usually not necessary. As they were after the first surgery, soft foods will be recommended until any tenderness subsides, but the time spent on a modified diet is typically shorter.

The one post-operative measure that doesn't change following second-stage surgery is hygiene. Though not nearly as stringent as the guidelines that followed your implant surgery, hygiene requirements again need to be followed thoroughly. Because the tissue around the surgical sites is likely to be tender and/or sensitive for up to ten days following the procedure, brushing around the surgical areas can be difficult, although normal brushing around the rest of your natural teeth should continue. Rinsing and buffing gently around the surgical sites with a Q-tip wetted with lukewarm water and/or a water/rinse solution is helpful. A combination of equal parts hydrogen peroxide, your favorite mouthwash, and water offers the added plus of foaming soft debris and foods away from your surgical sites. The same mixture of water with chlorhexidine or another anti-bacterial prescription mouth rinse adds the benefits of fighting the bacteria that can cause the formation of plaque with resultant infection.

Normal brushing usually can be resumed three to five days after the procedure along with the rest of your usual daily activities, exercise, and diet.

Checking In

Again, your doctor may want to see you a week or so after your second-stage surgery, to check on your progress, and perhaps on one or more subsequent dates until your healing is complete. When it is, you have entered the home stretch of your implant treatment.

Jean Friedman

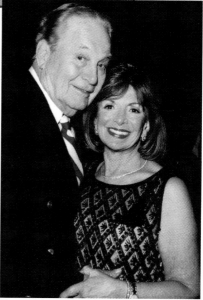

Most of my patients lead busy lives, but like Jean, a fashion buyer and businesswoman, they make time for implant treatment because it improves their quality of life.

Jean Friedman is committed to quality. It shows in the loving restoration of a landmark nineteenth-century building she and her husband turned into a gallery on the shores of Lake Erie. It is evident in the fine art and collectibles, the fine watches and jewelry the store offers.

It shows in the merchandise she personally selects for the family's department store during frequent buying trips to the fabled fashion district of Manhattan.

And it shows in the way she takes care of herself.

At 80, Jean works out regularly at a health club. A day doesn't pass without her sit-up routine. She dresses stylishly in up-to-date fashions. And she's very conscious of her teeth.

"I work with the public," she says. "I still work four to five days a week in the stores, and I'm in New York seven times a year on buying trips." Jean's buying specialty in the family business that now embraces all five of her grown children is women's fashion, a notoriously youthful field.

"I work with much younger people. In the fashion markets, everyone is 20 to 30 years old. If they're 40, they're old. I'm twice that. If I looked dowdy, nobody would pay attention to me. That's not for me."

The people Jean meets probably never guessed she wore a removable partial denture which replaced missing teeth on the right and left back sides of her lower jaw before her implant surgery in 1988. But Jean knew.

"I always smile," she says, "and I was always aware of them."

Jean ended up in a partial denture for a common reason among people who grew up before the era of widespread preventative and rehabilitative dental care: "If you had a toothache, or anything was wrong, they just pulled your tooth."

She never liked the false teeth. "I hated taking them out. I hated cleaning them. They weren't comfortable." All the same, she wore them for 20 years—until she learned about dental implants.

"One day I told my dentist how much I hated the partials, and he said, 'I have a very good friend and colleague who may be able to help you.' "

With her instinct for quality, it didn't take long for Jean to figure out that dental implants were a solution that fit her like a *haute couture* gown.

> **Jean Friedman:**
> *The implants changed my life. It was like getting my own teeth back. It made me feel like I used to be.*

Because her bones had shrunk very little, her implant treatment was straightforward. Two implants were placed on either side of her lower jaw, replacing the two natural teeth lost on each side so many years before. In place of the detested partial, she received new permanent fixed restorations that were indistinguishable to her—or anyone else—from the natural teeth beside them.

"They changed my life," she says about her implants. "It was like getting my own teeth back. It made me feel like I used to be."

It's hard to imagine how Jean "used to be" given the whirlwind she remains today. Besides her numerous New York buying trips and work in the family business, she continues staging an annual family Christmas celebration that entices 40 family members to drop in and 30 of them to sit down to a bountiful home-cooked meal.

For Jean, the commitment to quality never ends.

8 Your Beautiful New Teeth

Patients often approach implant treatment with a photograph of teeth they like and ask, "Will my teeth look exactly like this?"

The answer is "No," and you can be relieved that it is.

Think of the parking lot at a busy public place. Hundreds of cars may fill it, and no two are ever absolutely identical. The same is true of your new teeth. Implant-supported teeth are customized not only for your mouth but for your face. Their size, their shape, their coloration, their design must be matched to *you* and your personal characteristics.

That picture you carry to your doctor will provide helpful information about your hopes and ideals, but it can't be duplicated because the subject may not be "you"—even if the subject is you at an earlier age.

The Finish Line

The "finish line" of your implant treatment is known as the restorative phase. If your case has been carefully planned, this stage probably began long ago, possibly without you even noticing. In a team approach, your implant surgeon, restorative dentist, and/or dental laboratory will have exchanged ideas, records, and plans. These may have included photographs, x-rays, models, and other diagnostic information. Your team members consulted on your treatment plan long before your first implant was placed. But as the patient, you are likely to feel you've reached the restorative phase of your implant treatment when you first visit the doctor who will develop your final prosthesis (new teeth).

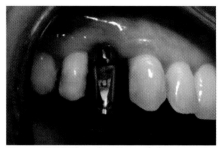

Figure 8.1 When healing of the gum tissue is complete, the healing abutment is replaced with the impression post.

Records

At this appointment and those following, several new records will be taken or ordered for use in building your final restoration. These typically include the following (Figures 8.1, 8.2):

- Preliminary impressions—a replica of any remaining natural teeth, your gums, and your implant abutments. The impression is made by placing an impression tray filled with a gel or putty in your mouth over the site being recorded.

- Bite relationship or incisal index—a record of the biting surface of your teeth which shows how the upper and lower jaws relate to one another when you bite. The index is obtained by placing a putty, gel, or wax-like wafer between your teeth and having you bite down on it.

- Study model—a cast that is made of both jaws complete with gums, teeth, and implant abutments. It is made from the impression in a very hard dental stone or plaster.

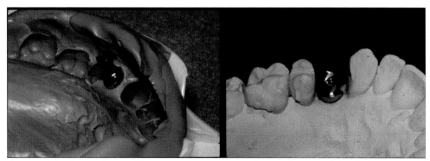

Figure 8.2 Once the mold, or impression, is obtained, a model of the jaw and implant is created in order to fabricate the tooth in the dental laboratory.

Communication

Your team members will use several methods for exchanging this information among themselves and sharing it with you. The doctor will send the photographs, impressions, and models described above to the laboratory. In turn, the lab will develop and deliver a series of mock-ups that your doctor will show you, try in your mouth, and eventually ask you to approve. If you are being restored with a single or multiple-tooth crown or bridge, the laboratory will send these items to your dentist for try-in and confirmation.

Artistic design

Dentistry is both science and art, and you will now become most keenly aware of the artistry involved in implant treatment.

A shade-guide system will be used to select a color for the teeth in your restoration that not only blends with adjacent and opposing teeth but also replicates the natural shading that occurs

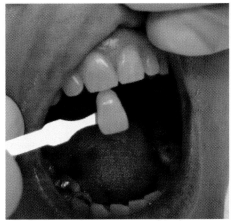

Figure 8.3 A shade guide is used to select the appropriate color of the teeth.

in your teeth from the gum lines to the biting edges. Sometimes, a dentist may even ask you to visit the dental laboratory so the technician building your teeth can be involved in the process of making the best possible match (Figure 8.3).

Additional artistic considerations are the size and shape of your teeth. Natural teeth come in a wide range of sizes. Shape varies, too, and can be oval, square, or rectangular. In those cases where both upper and lower jaws are being restored at the same time entirely with implants, the size and shape of the existing natural or prosthetic teeth in your mouth will be evaluated and used as guideposts for creating a replacement for the teeth that have been lost. When implants are being restored in only one jaw, the size and shape need to blend with the natural teeth or prosthesis that remains in the opposite jaw (Figure 8.4).

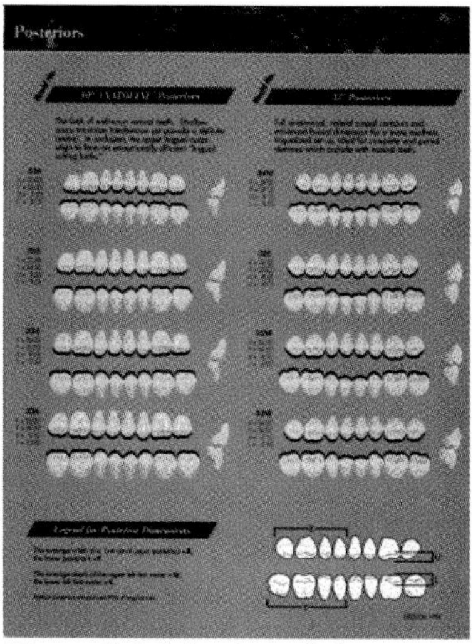

Your doctor may talk with you about tooth material. In the past, highly cosmetic porcelain was considered the ultimate restorative material. Today, new technology has expanded the choices to include space-age materials that provide highly aesthetic results. Some dentists and laboratories work exclusively or largely in one material or the other. Many will

Figure 8.4 Selection of the proper tooth size and shape is also important.

use porcelain on high-visibility teeth in the front of the mouth and more durable high-tech materials in the back of the mouth, where chewing exerts tremendous force. Material choices involve both artistic and scientific considerations.

There was a period of dental fashion when the goal of many patients was "piano keys"—a row of perfectly white, perfectly matched teeth. Increasingly dentists and patients alike seek a more natural look—teeth that may overlap a bit like the ones being replaced or teeth that are less than blinding white.

Once the teeth have been designed in size, shape, and arrangement, the laboratory may be asked to prepare a model of your final restoration. With these trial teeth in your mouth, you will be asked to evaluate tooth shape, size, configuration, how the bite feels, and all the other esthetic and functional aspects of your proposed new teeth.

This is the time to fine-tune!

Changes and adjustments still can be made easily while your restoration is in the trial state. In fact, the model teeth can be such an accurate predictor of the final outcome of treatment that your doctor may ask you to confirm your acceptance of it in writing.

You don't have your new teeth yet, but you know exactly how they will look and work. Ideally, when friends and family see you after treatment is complete, they will give you a puzzled stare and say, "You know, you really look good. There's something different, but I'm not sure what it is. Is it your makeup? Did you change your hair? Are you getting more sleep?"

This is the artistry we're all after—the subtle change that shows without announcing itself with a 32-piece orchestra. These, too, are issues that your restorative dentist will raise and discuss with you.

Timing

How long is the home stretch to the finish line?

Again, just as no one implant works in every site, no single answer addresses every patient. A simple case involving one or a few implants can be completed in several weeks to months. Some extremely complex cases take as long as a year or more.

In addition to the clinical demands of the case, patient scheduling can be a factor. When multiple appointments for diagnostics and try-ins are necessary but a patient travels frequently and can't always get to the dental office when the restoration is ready for evaluation, the duration of treatment may be extended.

However short or long the restorative stage, there comes a day when your final new teeth are finished. At long last, you can greet the world with a confident smile (Figures 8.5A-H).

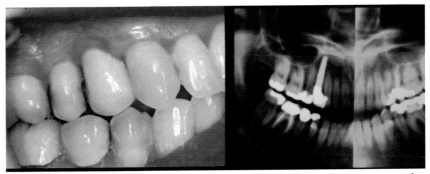

Figure 8.5A The final tooth crown has been attached to the implant, as seen in this picture and x-ray.

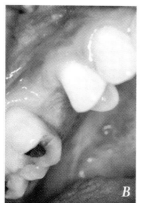

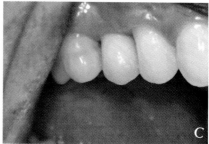

Figures 8.5B,C Before and after picture of a single-tooth implant.

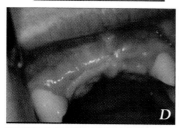

Figures 8.5D,E Before and after views of three implant-supported teeth, following a diving/ swimming accident.

Figure 8.5F Final x-rays of the case above.

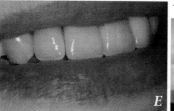

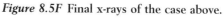

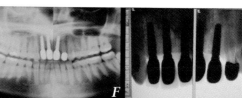

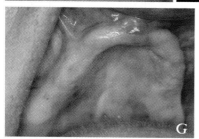

Figure 8.5G An upper jaw after all the teeth had been extracted and years of bone shrinkage had occurred.

Figure 8.5Ha,b The final result of the upper jaw implant reconstruction.

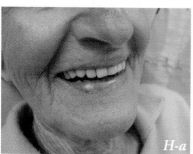

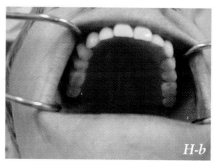

Bonnie Hotchkin

As an artist, Bonnie was highly attuned to the artistry of implant dentistry. She worked closely with me and her restorative dentist to assure that her new teeth would appear both beautiful and natural.

Bonnie Hotchkin was leaving a dermatology appointment when her physician popped the unexpected question.

"Bonnie," she asked. "Have you had a face lift?"

Bonnie's voice crackles with laughter as she recalls the episode.

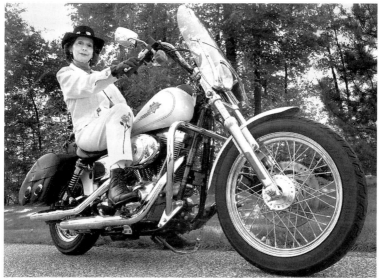

" 'Good heavens!' I said to her. 'You're a doctor. You should be able to tell that I haven't.' The doctor insisted. 'But you look so good.' "

Once a teenage fashion model and southern Missouri media personality who vowed all her life never to undergo plastic surgery, the 68-year-old artist has an explanation for her doctor's confusion.

"I think it was the implants," she confides.

Bonnie lost all her teeth to neglect and periodontal disease at the age of 29. "My husband at the time was in the military," she says. "Back then, you couldn't get free dental care. Well, we were poor as church mice, living from month to month, and I wasn't a good dental patient to begin with. I'd been traumatized as a child by a dentist who was downright vicious, and it left me with this terrible fear of dentistry.

"I didn't go to the dentist for years. If you didn't have money, you didn't get dental care anyway. By the time I finally went again, things had gotten so bad that the cost of fixing everything was just beyond us. 'You need to have all your teeth pulled,' the dentist said. So I did. We had to borrow money from the bank to get it done, but it seemed at the time like the only choice I had."

> **Bonnie Hotchkin:**
> *I tell my dentist he ought to tell people, "Skip the face lift. Come get your teeth done instead."*

Unlike many people, Bonnie didn't mind wearing dentures. After years of fighting gum disease, she loved the feeling that her mouth was clean and infection-free. The speech and eating problems experienced by many denture wearers never affected her. "Hardly anybody even knew I wore dentures. When I met the man I've been married to almost 20 years now, I asked if he could tell, and he said he couldn't, that he only thought my teeth might be capped because they were so perfect."

All the same, when her husband—"an engineer and a big reader"—began coming across articles about dental implants and sharing them with her, Bonnie was intrigued.

"The thing I didn't like was the way the dentures 'floated' on my gums, especially as I lost more bone and my gums became flatter," she says. "Sometimes when I sneezed or laughed real hard, I could feel them move around. They were mobile. Implants sounded so much more solid." And then there were the cosmetic benefits. "After 30 years without teeth, I had lost a lot of bone. The last time they remade my lower denture, they found that I'd lost a third or more of my remaining bone." As bone is lost, the face tends to sink inward. Because implants act like natural teeth roots to stop bone shrinkage, Bonnie learned they could also arrest or vastly slow the unpleasant cosmetic side effects of bone loss, an attractive additional benefit.

Bonnie made an appointment to find out more about implants, and a little more than two months later, treatment began. Because of the severity of her bone loss, both her upper and lower jawbones were rebuilt with bone grafts as part of the treatment. She decided to keep the denture in her upper jaw, where security tends to be less of an issue for denture wearers, but had four implants placed in her lower jaw. Ever the nervous dental patient, she underwent the surgery under a general anesthetic in an outpatient surgery center, a choice that is often offered to implant patients.

"There was *no way* I could have done this awake," she says with a new burst of laughter. "I am *still* not a good dental patient."

Bonnie's implants were restored with a removable clip-bar overdenture, another choice she felt strongly about. "The removable prosthesis was important to me," she says. "I didn't want to lose that feeling of cleanliness I enjoyed with the dentures."

Her new teeth even survived an unplanned test of durability. The proud owner and driver of a pinstriped Harley Davidson, Bonnie passed out from hypothermia shortly after she first learned to ride a motorcycle at the age of 63. "I knew it was cold, but I didn't realize what was happening," she recalls. After falling from the cycle, she bounced off two cars before landing with all her bones—and every one of her teeth—sound as ever.

Bonnie says she would recommend implants to anyone with tooth loss. Even though she never suffered from the problems that plague so many denture wearers, she says implants give her a stability the dentures never did.

And then there's that cosmetic bonus.

"I tell my dentist he ought to tell people, "Skip the face lift! Come get your teeth done instead!" In Bonnie Hotchkin's case, even her physician couldn't tell the difference.

9 *Living With Implants*

On the day you finally walk out of your doctor's office with your beautiful new teeth, *you* become the single most important member of your dental implant team.

Like natural teeth, dental implants require thorough, daily maintenance, and only you can provide it. Given the care they need, your implants can provide a lifetime of comfort, cosmetics, and reliable function. Neglected, they can be threatened by all the same troubles that undermine natural teeth when they're not properly maintained.

Sound routine maintenance is the proverbial ounce of prevention. In exchange for the few minutes a day required, you can:

- Prevent gum infection and/or disease (peri-implantitis)
- Prevent bone loss
- Prevent bad breath
- Prevent discomfort or pain
- Vastly increase the likelihood of lasting implant success
- Increase and maintain your quality of life, including your ease and enjoyment of eating, speaking, and smiling

Basic is Best

When it comes to implants, dentists like to say that basic hygiene is the best hygiene. A good routine of oral hygiene involves these daily measures:

Brushing

Dental plaque is a medium for bacteria and subsequent infection. When plaque is allowed to accumulate on your teeth, posts, clip-bar, prosthesis, or anywhere else in your mouth, you have opened the door to the potential for infection. Brushing is your first line of defense against this risk. Start by selecting a brush with soft, rounded bristles and an approved toothpaste. Use these to brush (Figure 9.1):

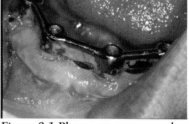

Figure 9.1 **Plaque on connector bar due to poor brushing, flossing, and home care techniques.**

- any remaining natural teeth
- your prosthesis, including the teeth and the inside and outside of the denture plate
- the abutments that protrude through your gums
- the gums themselves

Brush in the morning, after every meal, and before you go to bed. Because bacterial plaque builds up while you are asleep and the natural cleaning effect of saliva diminishes, brushing before you go to bed and first thing in the morning is particularly important (Figure 9.2). Supplemental brushing with a straight or cone-shaped interdental brush known as a proxabrush makes it easier to keep hard-to-reach spots clean. The proxabrush is particularly useful for reaching

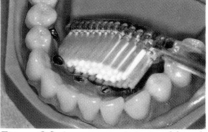

Figure 9.2 **An appropriate toothbrush should be selected just as it is for cleaning natural teeth.**

into the narrow spaces between implant posts and between your gum and the bottom of a fixed appliance. It can also be used to clean the underside of a fixed appliance. Proxabrushes are available in a purse or pocket-sized travel version, which is handy when you are out for meals or traveling (Figures 9.3A,B).

Brushing with either your regular toothbrush or an interdental brush offers the added benefit of stimulating your gums, which helps keep them healthy.

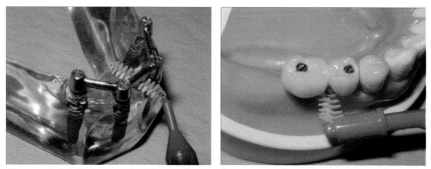

Figures 9.3A,B A proxabrush can be used in areas where there is limited access.

Flossing

Flossing cleans areas that even meticulous brushing can't reach. For your natural teeth, floss with the product you've always used. To floss your posts and/or bar, a woven or braided floss is particularly effective. Some of these come with threaders to help you maneuver the floss around bridgework or connector bars. Even cotton ribbon or yarn will work. The key is to use an effective product *with which you are comfortable*. If you find the "best" product in the world difficult to use, chances are you won't use it. Your hygienist or doctor can help you select a product you'll like.

Starting at one side of your mouth and working to the other, thread the floss around the back of each post so you can hold one end of the strand in each hand. Then use a shoeshine motion to polish the back, the sides, and finally the front of these posts. If you have a clip bar, perform the same procedure on the bar itself. Don't forget to floss the underside of the bar as well as the top and sides.

If you wear a fixed prosthesis, the floss can be used to scrub the underside of the prosthesis after brushing (Figures 9.4A,B).

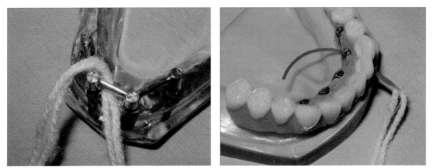

Figures 9.4A,B Either yarn or floss with a threader can be used in a "shoe shine" manner to assist in cleaning various areas of the implant(s) and crown(s).

Rinsing

Rinsing your mouth after brushing and flossing removes bacteria and any debris you have dislodged. An anti-bacterial product such as a chlorohexidine solution can provide additional protection against bacteria that like to breed in your mouth. You can also dip your proxabrush or a Q-tip into a small cup of the rinse and apply it directly to your posts, bar, or gum tissues, or soak your removable appliance in a denture cleanser. You may spit out the chlorohexidine solution, but do not rinse.

Other tools

Some patients supplement or substitute regular manual brushing with battery-powered brushing. The results are so much better than manual brushing that this has become an increasingly popular option. Patients with medical conditions that affect their manual dexterity (arthritis, carpel tunnel syndrome, Parkinson's disease, and/or stroke, for example) may find the automated toothbrush particularly helpful. Interchangeable brush tips that come with some automatic brushes make it easier to clean different problem areas in your mouth (Figure 9.5).

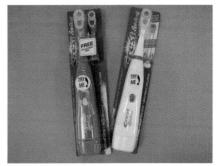

Figure 9.5 A variety of battery-operated toothbrushes are now on the market. The "Spinbrush" has proven to be extremely beneficial for a good home program of oral hygiene.

An oral irrigation system can be helpful in removing plaque and debris after cleaning but should be used with extreme care to avoid traumatizing the tissues. Water flow should always be set at the lowest possible level and directed away from the gum tissue.

Time

The entire cleaning process takes less than a hair or makeup routine or a shave and regular brushing—a small investment in exchange for protecting the time, effort, and dollars you have invested in your new teeth.

Might is NOT Right

Even though your implant posts and bar are metal, they can be scratched. Because scratches create a breeding ground for bacteria, it is important to avoid any tool or technique that may scratch your implant devices. Metal scalers, probes, or other tools should NEVER be used by

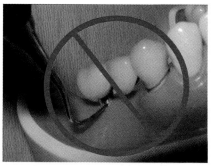

Figure 9.6 Metal instruments, such as scalers, should not be used on the metal surface of implants as they will leave scratches and cause a more rapid accumulation of debris on the implant surface.

you, the patient, around your implant posts, clip-bar, and/or attachments. Such tools can easily damage even the strongest metals and may set up a chain of events that can jeopardize your implant success (Figure 9.6).

Likewise, using unnecessary force while brushing or cleaning your teeth or gums can be harmful to the health of your implants, especially if you are using power brushes. Avoid sawing on your gums while flossing. As mentioned above, if a water-irrigation system is used, avoid a strong water flow or pointing the wand toward your gums.

When it comes to implant maintenance, the watchwords are *thorough* and *gentle*.

Monitoring

The vast majority of your implant maintenance consists of the daily habits already described. Two other habits will also promote the health of your implants.

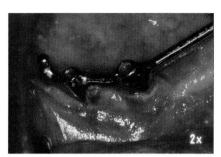

Figure 9.7 Swelling and unhealthy gum tissue due to poor oral hygiene.

Be observant

Your doctor and, eventually, your experience will teach you when all's well with your implants. The person in the best position to detect when it's not is you. Inspect your gums when you clean. Any bleeding when you brush or floss is abnormal. Angry redness or swelling

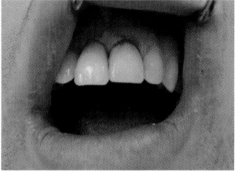

Figure 9.8 Bleeding of the unhealthy gum tissues due to poor daily oral hygiene.

of your gum tissues can also be a sign of infection. Pain or mobility in your implants is another indicator that something is probably amiss. When your home observation detects a potential problem, call your doctor immediately. Don't wait for your next scheduled appointment (Figures 9.7, 9.8).

Make and keep routine follow-up appointments

Two critical events take place at routine follow-up appointments with your implant doctor. One is that your posts, bar, and/or attachments and prosthesis are professionally cleaned by the doctor or hygienist. Even the best home care isn't able to remove all the plaque that a trained and equipped professional can remove. Just as your natural teeth need routine cleaning, so do your implant components. The second is that your doctor checks your bone, gums, soft tissues, and implant components for health and stability. Your bite is checked. Small emerging problems can be detected and treated before they have a chance to grow into big full-blown ones.

In the case of some implant-supported appliances, parts may need to be replaced periodically. Failure to do so can result in complications and/or failure of your prosthesis. Your routine appointments are when timely part replacements may be needed.

Beyond Maintenance

Beyond routine maintenance, here's what you can expect from your new life with dental implants:

- You *will* be able to eat the same diet you ate when all your natural teeth were intact. You may even be able to eat corn on the cob, peanuts, popcorn. You will *not* have to worry about your denture slipping when you laugh or clicking when you talk.
- You will *not* be troubled by sore spots from a moving, floppy denture plate on your gums.
- You will *not* have to worry about your denture falling into your martini glass or onto your dinner plate.
- If you replaced a denture, you will be able to throw away your glues and adhesives.
- Your quality of life will improve.

Commitment

In the months before you walk out of your doctor's office with your beautiful new teeth, one or more dentists, dental assistants, laboratory technicians, and maybe others will have worked long and hard to address the personal

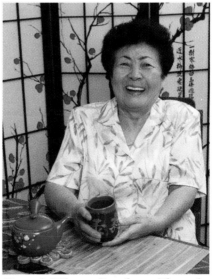

Figure 9.9 The quality of your life can be increased with dental implants and a good daily oral hygiene program.

needs, wants, and desires you identified at your very first appointment. With the achievement of these goals, you can expect to enjoy them for a long time provided you play your role.

Living successfully with dental implants requires *your* commitment to be an active, dedicated member of your implant team. Fulfill your part as diligently as the other team members have fulfilled theirs, and your future will be as bright as your new smile (Figure 9.9).

SUCCESS STORY:

Myrtle Watson

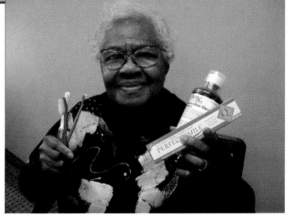

I always tell my patients that they are the most important member of their implant team. Myrtle's story explains why.

After 30 years of teaching, Myrtle Watson knows that

Figure 9.10 Myrtle Watson with all of her oral home-care equipment

good students follow directions carefully. It's a conviction she brings to her life with dental implants.

"I firmly believe in cooperating with the doctors," she says with the authority of a veteran schoolteacher. "I figure this: They're the experts. They're the ones who went to school to learn how to take care of us. I expect them to do it. But if I don't do my part, then I have only myself to blame."

Myrtle is especially attuned to the importance of good oral hygiene because of the history that led up to her implant surgery in 1988.

Though a stickler for good health practices, poor dental hygiene early in her life led to gum disease. By her 30s, Myrtle's gums had receded so severely that her teeth were becoming loose.

"My dentist remarked one day when I told him the teeth were getting loose, 'Oh, well, we might as well pull them because you're going to lose them anyway.' Which was *bad* advice. I changed dentists.

"The new one sent me to a periodontist who might have helped me if I'd come to him sooner. I could tell he wanted to help so much, but it was a little too late." The teeth couldn't be saved. Before 40, Myrtle was wearing full upper and lower dentures.

For some years, she lived happily with dentures. But as the bone beneath her gums shrank without tooth roots to maintain it, there was less and less structure to support the plates. They became increasingly uncomfortable. Eventually, chewing even a banana was painful.

That's when she opted for dental implants. In late 1988 at the age of 68, Myrtle was treated with four implants in the front of her lower jaw. After the sites had healed, she was restored with a clip-bar removable overdenture.

"There was a great and immediate improvement," she says, "because I could chew again." She also was able to overcome a small nagging fear that her worst moment as a denture wearer—when her plate fell out while she was talking—might be repeated.

Myrtle's loss of her natural teeth taught her that small problems can grow into big and irreversible ones if they aren't detected and treated promptly, so she keeps her annual recall appointments and any interim check-ups without fail.

Myrtle Watson:

When I go to my implant check-ups, I'm not doing my doctor a favor. I'm doing myself a favor. There is no reason implants shouldn't last the rest of my life, but that requires taking care of them. If anything happens to my implants what am I going to do then? I can't wear dentures. It would be awful. I would just die.

"When I get my implants checked, I'm not doing my doctor a favor. I'm doing myself a favor," she says. "There's no reason that implants shouldn't last the rest of my life, but that requires taking care of them. If anything happens to my implants, what am I going to do then? I can't wear dentures. It would be awful. I would just die!"

She may no longer be the schoolteacher she was for 30 years, but Myrtle proves she's a good student every single day, year after year.

10 *When Things Go Wrong*

To Ella Mae Shaker, implants seemed like a fairytale solution to a lifelong torment.

"I always had very bad teeth, even as a kid," says the cheerful, 71-year-old office worker. As a young women, she lost teeth every time she got pregnant—and she was pregnant six times. By 39, she retained only six teeth in her lower jaw. "I can remember my dentist saying to me, 'Treasure these teeth because you will never be able to wear a full denture.' The bone there was knife-thin."

She tried to safeguard her remaining lower teeth. But several eventually fell victim to irreparable decay. Her finances seemed too limited to allow her to undergo implant therapy. That's when fate intervened. Employed as a secretary in the Department of Oral and Maxillofacial Surgery at Mt. Sinai Medical Center in Cleveland, Ella Mae learned about a patient study that was getting underway. She volunteered to participate and was accepted. In May of 1995, the remaining teeth in her lower jaw were extracted. She received five implants that ultimately supported a connector bar and overdenture, and she prepared to live with her new teeth happily ever after.

But Ella Mae's tale has had a few extra chapters.

"I've had some little complications along the way," Ella Mae discloses. Things have gone wrong that she did not anticipate.

Several infections plagued one spot in her mouth intermittently. Five years after the initial implant surgery, she began feeling pain in the area where she'd had the infections, and an x-ray revealed that the bone around the implant had receded.

Although most patients never have any problems with their implants, a minority, like Ella Mae, encounter some kind of problem. When this occurs, their stories need not take a tragic turn. Most of the time, problems that develop in the wake of implant reconstruction can be resolved. The key is to address them swiftly and conscientiously.

Let's take a look at just what can go wrong with dental implants and how these events are managed.

Soft-Tissue Problems

Like natural teeth, implants are surrounded by gum tissue that must be cared for properly. But some people don't follow these instructions. When debris builds up in their mouths, the tissue around the implants can become inflamed and swollen. Eventually, it may bleed when brushed; sometimes something as simple as eating salad or crusty bread can injure or further irritate the fragile tissue. The condition in which the gum tissue around the implants becomes tender and sore is known as gingivitis or peri-implantitis (Figure 10.1).

Poor hygiene is not the only cause. Ella Mae, for example, worked hard to follow her doctor's directions. But she has always healed poorly, she reports.

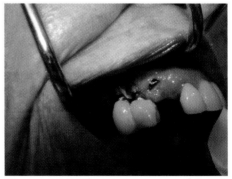

Figure 10.1 The appearance of "peri-implantitis" with swelling, debris, and overall unhealthy tissues.

She recalls how her earlobes failed to heal for years after she had them pierced—a simple procedure from which most people quickly recover. "I think it's just something in my body," she suggests.

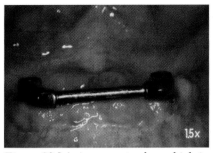

Figure 10.2A A connector bar which is too close to the gum tissue and will not allow for proper cleaning.

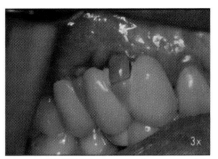

Figure 10.2B The space between this patient's teeth is not open enough to allow for proper cleaning with a brush, proxabrush, or floss. Infection is likely to result.

For other patients, the design of the restoration may inadvertently lead to trouble. If contoured incorrectly, the prosthesis may cause an area of the gums to be inaccessible for cleaning. Plaque and calculus then build up, and tenderness and inflammation may result.

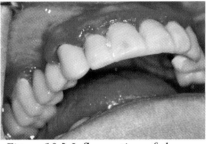

Figure 10.3 Inflammation of the gum tissue.

This in turn can create a vicious circle: patients are likely to avoid brushing these areas of soreness—which of course only makes the problem worse (Figures 10.2A,B; 10.3).

If the design of the prosthesis prevents a patient from cleaning some area of the gums, the doctor may be able to fix the problem by reshaping and repolishing the prosthesis. In rare instances, the restoration may have to be remade altogether.

When inadequate hygiene is the culprit, a number of steps may be necessary. A thorough cleaning of the abutment and prosthesis often suffices to relieve the irritated tissue. Sometimes learning the hard way about the consequences of poor hygiene is all it takes to change a patient's ways. Periodic follow-up visits, which may include sessions with a hygienist, can also reinforce how critical it is that implants be cleaned properly. If the tissue deterioration is advanced, deeper cleaning and scaling and a course of antibiotics are sometimes required. In the worst instances, when infection has caused the gum tissue to recede around the implant neck, the doctor may recommend soft-tissue grafting.

On some of the occasions when Ella Mae's gum became infected, she was given a course of oral and/or local antibiotics to bring the tissues back to health. But after several years, she began feeling a different sort of pain in the area, and an x-ray revealed that bone loss had occurred around the implant.

Hard-Tissue Problems

Whatever the cause of peri-implantitis, it may progress to the point where it affects the jawbone underlying the gum. The chronic irritation and infection of the gums can cause the bone to deteriorate.

Mechanical factors also can make this happen. It's extremely important that the teeth come together in a way that distributes force evenly throughout the mouth. If for some reason this "bite relationship" is not correct and too much pressure is applied in one spot, the consequences can be damaging. It's a little like driving a car down a badly maintained road. If the vehicle keeps bouncing over potholes, pretty soon the shock absorbers and springs will deteriorate. Bone is similar. Chronic assault can make the bone around the implant dissolve.

Sometimes this happens right after the implant(s) and/or prostheses are placed. A design flaw in the prosthesis can result in a poor bite. When this occurs, the restoration or bite must be adjusted. On the other hand, excessive pressure in one area of the mouth may not begin until months or years after osseointegration has occurred.

One patient may start grinding and clenching in response to increased stress in his or her life. Another might develop a bad habit such as chewing on pencils or clamping down on the stem of a pipe. These behaviors can harm the prosthesis, which in turn can harm the bone around an implant or implants. Sometimes accidents cause problems with one or both of the temperomandibular joints (TMJs). This, too, can create an uneven bite.

When bone loss around an implant does occur, what happens next will depend upon a couple of factors. If only a small amount of bone has disappeared from around the top of the implant, it may not be necessary to do anything. As long as the body of the implant isn't moving and the doctor feels confident that the bone loss has stopped, close observation of the implant over time may be all that is required. When a significant amount of bone loss occurs, however, usually something must be done to prevent the implant from finally loosening in its socket. Ella Mae, for example, had lost about 60 percent of the bone around one of her implants. Although the implant was still firmly fixed in her jaw, her doctor recommended surgical intervention to assure the implant's continued health and stability. The tissue was opened up, and all the infected tissue around the implant was removed. A combination of platelet-rich plasma and bone-graft material was then applied over the area where the bone was missing. The implant is still in place and functioning well (Figures 10.4A,B).

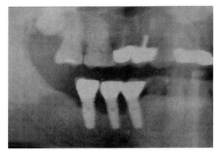

Figure 10.4A The x-ray shows loss of bone around the implants due to lack of proper home care and routine follow-up visits to the doctor for periodic cleaning and evaluation.

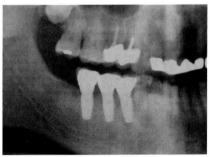

Figure 10.4B On this x-ray, improved bone fill can clearly be seen after appropriate treatment with a bone graft and platelet-rich plasma.

On rare occasion, replacing the implant may be necessary. Sometimes this is combined with additional bone grafting, but in other instances, it's sufficient to remove the loose implant and replace it with a larger-diameter one. As always, the quality and quantity of bone dictates which course must be followed.

Accidental Damage

Accidents happen. When they do, they can damage implants and fixed or removable prostheses that have been functioning well for years and even decades. It's easy to understand, for example, how a car crash or a fall can fracture a prosthetic tooth or overdenture. Like any structure, artificial teeth are vulnerable to sudden impact. Even a rear-end collision and resulting whiplash can break a prosthesis as the lower jaw snaps against the upper jaw. Sometimes a much more mundane action can wreak havoc. A patient bites on a nut or chomps down on a piece of gristle, and the prosthesis chips, cracks, or breaks. If this happens, quick professional attention can limit the damage and inconvenience. In many instances, the existing prosthesis can be professionally repaired, though sometimes replacement will be necessary (Figure 10.5).

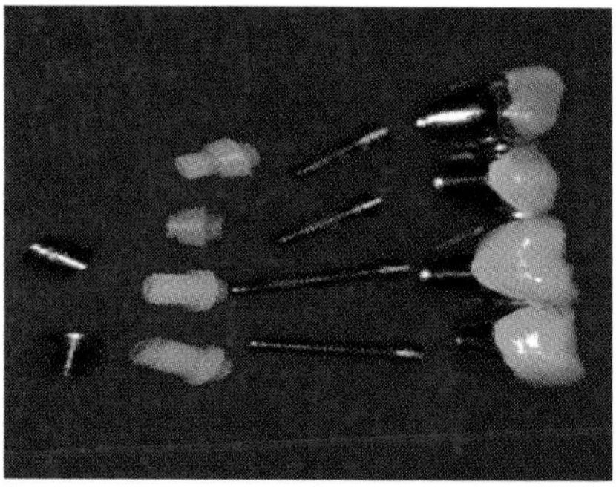

Figure 10.5 An accident caused multiple fractures of the implants and components. All were repaired.

Under no circumstances should a patient repair a broken prosthesis at home. People sometimes attempt to do this, using Super Glue or some other bonding agent. While they might succeed in joining the broken pieces together, it's very difficult, if not impossible, for a non-professional to ensure that the bite is correct and that no undue pressure is being placed upon the underlying implants, gum, or jawbone.

At the other end of the spectrum, some patients don't realize that their prostheses have broken. This can occur when the fracture is a small one, invisible to the untrained eye. Such a break can cause micromovement that eventually damages the bone. Imagine holding the top of a fence post and shaking it very gently over time. Eventually, the place where the fence post enters the ground will become enlarged. Micromovement can cause the same thing to happen to the implant.

One other category of prosthetic problem causes micromovement fairly commonly: a loosening (rather than breakage) of the prosthesis. The screw securing a fixed-removable denture may loosen microscopically. With a cemented prosthesis, the cement seal can sometimes wash out. In either case, the prosthesis will stay in place, but tiny movements over time take their toll on the underlying implant(s).

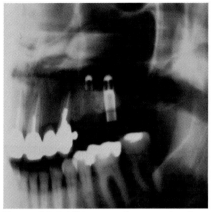

Figure 10.6 This x-ray shows an implant that fractured as a result of prolonged micromovement of the prosthesis. The patient failed to return to the doctor for routine care, which might have prevented the fracture.

If bone breakdown occurs and becomes excessive, several things can happen. Any implant that becomes mobile will need to be replaced. In rare cases, the screw that holds the abutment in place or even the implant itself can fracture (Figure 10.6).

How does any patient know that damage to the prosthesis or bone loss has occurred?

Often the patient's earliest clue will be swollen or bleeding gums, pain, or a loose restoration. However, by the time something begins to hurt, a serious problem has usually occurred. That's why it's so important instead to return to the dentist for periodic appointments. The combination of the professional examinations and x-rays allows most problems to be detected long before any symptoms develop. If too much time has not elapsed between visits and the level of home care is good, prompt intercession can reverse most problems—before they become painful, expensive, and time-consuming.

Medical and Dental Complications

Medical and unrelated dental problems that develop after the implant treatment is complete can also cause problems for implant patients. Some individuals develop severe uncontrolled diabetes, for example. This disease can make the body more prone to infection. If a person's level of oral hygiene is only fair, breakdown of the soft tissue and subsequent bone loss may occur. Or a patient may develop cancer and require chemotherapy or radiation. Such treatment can compromise the immune system in general and also can cause ulcers and/or irritate the soft tissue in the mouth. Tooth-brushing becomes painful, the patient becomes less diligent about maintenance, and the cycle of deterioration unfolds.

Yet another example of this sort of problem is the patient who develops a connective tissue disease (such as erythema multiforme, lichen planus, lupus erythematosus, or pemphigus). Such individuals are prone to developing oral lesions and ulcers and cannot manage their oral hygiene as well.

If a dental problem develops in the area adjacent to an implant, it too can spell trouble for the implant in rare cases, as you will read in the following Success Story.

Who Pays?

To avoid misunderstanding and unhappiness, all implant patients should discuss with their doctors before treatment begins what will happen if anything goes wrong. Who will bear the financial responsibility of correcting any problems that develop?

If an implant or prosthesis breaks shortly after placement, and the damage was due to a design flaw, most practitioners will absorb the cost of replacing the broken item. A few doctors offer a blanket guarantee. On the other hand, problems that develop years later or because of the patient's failure to return for periodic exams and follow recommended hygiene routines are almost always considered to be the patient's responsibility.

A large gray area falls between these two extremes. Understanding the doctor's policy in advance can prevent bad feelings in the future. Yet another form of insurance against disappointment is to realize that biological systems are complex and sometimes unpredictable. Moreover, implants are artificial substitutes for God-given body parts, so there can be no absolute guarantees.

With patience and commitment, however, problems can be overcome. That's the attitude expressed by Ella Mae Shaker, when reflecting on her experience. "Things happen," she says. "I was never discouraged even when I had some problems. I just kind of trudged through them because I was so appreciative of what was going on. In my case, implants were a salvation."

Marscee Wolkis

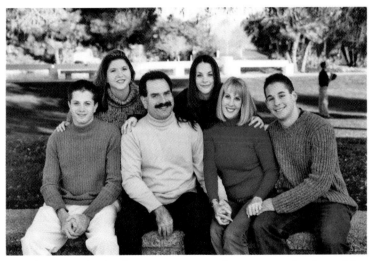

An often-overlooked consequence of some medical problems is their impact on teeth and bone. My patient Marscee learned this early in life.

"I hate people who have good teeth," Marscee Wolkis jokes. When she flashes a gleaming set of perfectly straight teeth, her comment seems perplexing, but then she explains. "What I really mean is that I'm envious of people with naturally good teeth. I wasn't that lucky."

Misfortune befell Marscee at the age of 15. One day, her mother noticed that she was limping. She determined that her daughter hadn't been involved in any accidents then took Marscee to the family doctor. Tests revealed a tumor on the girl's hip, and further investigation showed it to be the result of chronic osteomyelitis, a disease that slowly eats away at bones. Unless caught early, it can eventually cripple its victims and limit their physical activities.

Fortunately for Marscee, a surgeon was able to remove the tumor. And the operation yielded more good news: the growth was benign. But additional trouble for the girl soon surfaced—this time in the form of a tumor within her jaw.

"In one jaw surgery, they took out a large piece of the bone," Marscee recalls. "In another, they had to scrape from the right to the left portion of the jaw." In the process, Marscee had to have four of her permanent teeth removed from the right side of her lower jaw.

Marscee Wolkis:

Implant surgery was like the last step in getting my life together after my illness.

Around this time, she and her parents learned of an experimental treatment involving hyperbaric oxygen that had apparently cured other patients with chronic osteomyelitis. Eager to put her disease forever behind her, Marscee and her parents decided she should travel to an Air Force base in San Antonio, Texas, where she could receive the treatments. During the course of several lengthy stays, Marscee underwent a series of "dives" in the hyperbaric chamber. Each time, she had to sit quietly, breathing pure oxygen pressurized to a depth of 100 feet. The hope was that the effects of the pure oxygen would reverse the disease and disintegrate any incipient new tumors.

The treatments were a stunning success. "After that, I never had another problem," Marscee says. By the time she celebrated her 19th birthday, all evidence of the disease had disappeared. Because her physician believed that a warm, dry climate might help prevent a recurrence, Marscee moved to Arizona, where she enjoyed an active college life. These were happier times than her years in high school had been, when illness had clouded her future. Yet in college, Marscee felt depressed by one reminder of her recent tribulation.

Although a partial denture filled the gap in her mouth where the tumor had been removed, the false teeth embarrassed her. "I was never, ever comfortable with the denture," Marscee explains. "I would smile or laugh, and in a split second, I'd remember that I had this fake partial. I felt it shone like a beacon every time I opened my mouth."

When she fell in love and got engaged, she shrank from telling her fiancé about her denture. Only as their wedding day approached did she break the news to him. "He laughed!" she recalls. "He said something like, 'Are you kidding?' He couldn't have cared less about it."

Despite his understanding, Marscee continued to feel insecure. "I'll never forget having to take the partial out and clean it. Or worrying about it when I smiled. Sometimes food got caught underneath it. Sometimes it would break," she recalls. She'd heard about dental implants, and a few years after her 30th birthday, she could wait no longer. "I was ready," she says. "I wanted something stable. I wanted something that looked real and felt real and would be stronger."

Over the course of the next few months, Marscee twice flew back to Cleveland in order to undergo surgeries. Chips of bone-grafting material were used to reshape her jaw and support the placement of four implants. The implants healed well and four beautiful reconstructed teeth were eventually connected to them.

Throughout all the treatment phases, Marscee's spirits remained high. "I had some minor discomfort when the implants were placed. But it wasn't anything like the original tumor surgery that I'd had done on my jaw," she says. "I did great. I was so excited that it was finally happening."

In the dozen years following her implant surgery, Marscee often expressed delight with the way her mouth looked and felt. "It was like the last step in getting my life together after my illness."

Some years later, Marscee developed a periodontal problem with the adjacent natural tooth. She ultimately underwent periodontal treatment that included tissue grafting and the use of a membrane to attempt regeneration around the natural tooth. But the infection spread to the bone around the adjacent implant, which eventually had to be removed. Fortunately, Marscee was able to continue functioning on the other implants in her mouth with the same prosthesis. When later jaw alignment problems arose that were unrelated to her implant treatment, she was able to undergo treatment for those with braces (orthodontia).

If her dental history has been more unusual than that of most people, Marscee shrugs and says, "It could have been a *lot* worse." She adds that her experience with implants has been a bright spot. In fact, since Marscee's implant treatment, her 65-year-old father has replaced most of his failing teeth with implants. "And now my mother is about to get them too."

11 The Future of Implants

The year is 2025. Your right front canine—the one for which you had the root canal so many years ago—has finally fractured, beyond repair. Fortunately, your dentist anticipated this and obtained precise measurements of the tooth before it broke.

Now he sends a fragment to a local bioengineering firm, where dental stem cells are quickly extracted from it. Within weeks, the biotechnicians have grown a replacement tooth made of your own genetic material. The structure is complex, including all the components in your original canine: crown, root, nerves, blood vessels.

Once the replacement tooth is ready, your oral surgeon removes the remaining portion of the original from your mouth. Then he implants the substitute, adding biological cement and other materials to guarantee it will bond quickly with the jawbone. Within weeks, the new tooth, as pristine as a schoolchild's, is ready to bite into the toughest piece of steak. Assuming it receives routine daily care, it will serve you well for the rest of your life.

Science fiction?

Well, yes. But the scenario isn't hard to imagine, in light of research that's already under way. In the fall of 2002, for example, scientists at the Forsyth Institute in Boston announced that they had used enzymes to isolate immature tooth cells from

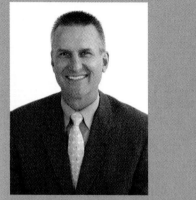
pigs. They implanted the cells in the stomachs of rats, close to a rich supply of blood. Within 30 weeks, small recognizable tooth crowns containing dentin and enamel had grown, leading the researchers to predict that human-tooth regeneration might be possible within 10 years.

A great deal of work remains before exact biological copies of our teeth can be routinely grown and transplanted. To put things in perspective, scientists have yet to determine *whether* dental stem cells even exist in humans, let alone to fine-tune the methods for growing perfect replacements from them.

All the same, some innovations already are dramatically reshaping implant dentistry, and more appear on the horizon every year. Here's a look at some of the most promising.

More Implant Doctors for More Patients

Only within the past two or three years have some dental schools begun including dental implant training in their curricula. More schools will follow suit, and as a result, more young general dentists will start their first practices trained to deliver implant therapy to their patients. This is a very different situation from the past when any dentist who wanted to offer implants needed to take time away from his or her practice and seek out specialized graduate-level or continuing-education training.

A greater number of these new implant doctors will be general dentists than is the case today. Their ranks vastly surpass those of the dental specialists who have provided the majority of implant treatment since implant dentistry joined the mainstream more than 40 years ago. As these plentiful general dentists begin to incorporate implants into their everyday practices, consumers choices will multiply.

This development couldn't be more timely. Although baby boomers are reaching their golden years with far more of their natural teeth than their forebears hung onto, the sheer number of these individuals and their expectations for a high quality of life suggest they will seek dental implant treatment in record numbers in the next 20 years.

Better Diagnosis, Better Tools, Better Parts

Implant patients are already enjoying breakthroughs in diagnostic technology and can look forward to more.

LOOKING FORWARD

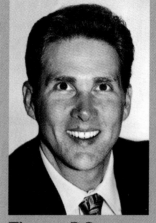

**Thomas P. Stratton,
Vice President and
General Manager
Friadent CeraMed Division
of Dentsply International**

The new frontier will be general dentists accepting implants as a part of everyday dentistry. And that's absolutely going to happen. As patients start learning about implant dentistry and obtaining second opinions, I think there will be a unified message: that implant dentistry is a viable form of treatment. The other thing we'll see is new ways of encouraging the hard and soft tissues to grow around the implants. Even though things work very well right now, there's still room for improvement.

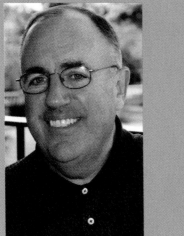

LOOKING FORWARD

**Bill Ryan, President
Straumann Implant Company**

Rather than one implant satisfying all situations, there will be more and more specialty implants. And then as we go further and further into the future, we'll see the implants themselves becoming delivery systems for growth factors and even therapeutics. In other words, the implant will not only replace the tooth but also provide a continuous supply of localized medicine such as antibiotics. I also believe that more and more expertise will be incorporated into the computerized planning and guidance systems that help the doctors. Doctors will always be needed, but robots may, in 10 years or so, be developed enough to handle simple surgical procedures, thus freeing the doctors for higher-level activities.

Doctors have begun using digital radiographs, for example, to obtain an instant computer image of what's going on beneath the patient's gums. These x-rays don't have to be developed in a darkroom, and they can be retaken on the spot if necessary. Besides providing diagnostic information faster than ever before, they reduce patient radiation exposure by 85 percent. What's more, the doctor can manipulate these images in an integrated office-computer system to increase the useful information they provide.

Ultrasound technology for dentistry also is emerging. One Israeli company has developed a way to use ultrasound on the jawbone, dispensing with radiation altogether. Ultrasound can also be used as a navigational guide during surgery. This innovation would make it easier to avoid vital structures near implant sites, reposition nerves, and otherwise refine implant surgery.

Implants and their attachments may evolve further as well, becoming so customized that the shape of each would be determined by the anatomy of the patient and the site where it was being placed.

Biological Breakthroughs

Implant futurists dream of an array of bioengineering advances that will enhance the success of implant treatment even beyond its current impressive levels.

The use of platelet-rich plasma derived from a patient's own blood supply already is changing the nature of implant dentistry. When this biochemical elixir is applied to fresh surgical sites, it decreases inflammation and swelling, enhance wound closure, accelerate bone growth, and reduce overall healing time.

For the future, most of the dental industry leaders featured in this chapter envision that more bioactive substances will be developed, and the substances will be delivered in exciting new ways. They may be built into implant coatings, for example, so that tissue adheres better, eliminating the minimal bone and gum loss that sometimes occurs. Or they may be incorporated into biological cements that will stabilize implants in even the worst bone.

As genetic data becomes easier to collect and analyze, futurists say implant treatment may eventually be refined to accommodate every individual's personal body chemistry and genetic codes.

LOOKING FORWARD

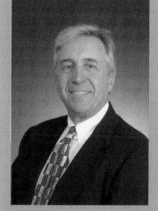

**John Kay, Ph. D.,
Vice President of Research
and Development
GenSci Orthobiologics**

It may be 20 years out, but doctors may someday be able to customize every implant surgery to match the patient's own genetics. You'll be able to determine in advance if a patient is genetically disposed to poor bone healing, for example. For the patient who is, the doctor may be able to take extra steps to counteract the genetic handicap. People who once would not have qualified for implant therapy will be able to take advantage of all the benefits that implants offer.

LOOKING FORWARD

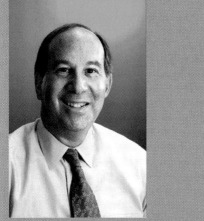

Bob Salvin, President and Chief Executive Officer Salvin Dental Specialties

Patients are going to live longer. If someone born today were to buy life insurance, the life expectancy table would be 110 years. Longevity encourages people to invest more in feeling and looking better. I think the bottom line is that dental implant procedures will become as common and as readily accepted as cataract procedures are now. Just as people are getting a second set of eyes by having cataract surgeries, they're also going to demand a third set of teeth. I also see practices transforming themselves into dental implant centers, much like ophthalmologists have transformed their practices into Lasik centers.

Shorter Treatment Times

As discussed earlier in the book, implant treatment has already begun to evolve from multiple procedures that take place over an extended period of time to fewer ones that culminate in earlier tooth restoration. The appeal of a shorter treatment span is not lost on dental clinicians or the manufacturers who supply them. A number of techniques and products that shorten treatment time have already emerged. More can be expected.

Patients who today are not candidates for immediate tooth replacement may tomorrow qualify as technological innovations that are dreams now become realities. The day may come when few patients pass even a single day following implant surgery without new teeth. Many in implant dentistry believe shorter treatment times will become the norm.

Implants as a Routine

At the outset of this book, we talked about the days when dental implants were a fringe activity in dentistry. Happily for hundreds of thousands of patients, those days are long gone. As Marty Dymek of Nobel Biocare says,

"The good news with dental implants is that the materials and procedures we have today are incredibly reliable, incredibly resilient, and meet the vast majority of patient needs. We don't have to wait for any huge breakthroughs in technology."

As good as the news is, all indications are that it will be even better in the future.

Adds Dymek, "The work we've done over the past 10 to 15 years has already positioned implants to be far more accepted, far more routine, and far more a part of everyday dentistry as we move into the twenty-first century."

LOOKING FORWARD

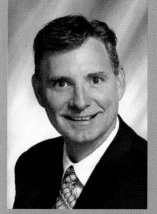

Gary Tureski, President Harvest Technologies

A growing emphasis in surgery is the use of biologics to enable the body to heal in a natural but accelerated manner. Proteins are the key, but there may be hundreds of thousands to several million different proteins. Recent research has indicated that there may even be distinct differences in proteins from person to person. One of our emerging technologies enables the clinician to harvest the patient's own unique healing proteins, intact and completely bioactive, for immediate application to the wound site. We are just beginning to understand the role these important proteins can play, but we know they offer a safe, cost-effective means of accelerating healing naturally.

LOOKING FORWARD

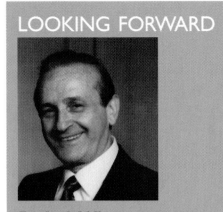

**Dr. Jack Wimmer,
President and Director
Park Dental
Research Corporation**

How far we have come from the pioneering days of dental implantology! Today many practitioners place dental implants, and the vast majority of both professionals and patients are very pleased with the results. In the future, we will advance much farther. Dental implants will be made of non-metallic materials. Computer and laser-enhanced placement techniques will become commonplace. Implants will become a routine part of dentistry, with such a high level of acceptance and predictability that all dental practitioners will offer this service to the public.

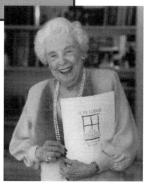

As implant technology continues to improve, it will serve more and more patients like Jeanette. For the time being, she's my oldest patient.

Jeanette Silber's personal physician once asked her what age she would choose if she could be younger. She didn't hesitate. "Eighty-five," she told him, with a twinkle in her eye. "Why not?" the 100-year-old elaborates. "I don't take any medication. I'm out at nine in the morning, and I'm busy all day. I've done volunteer work for practically every charity in Cleveland." A heavy schedule of meetings and activities continues to keep her on the run.

Growing old could be hard at times, Jeanette admits. But "I like a challenge," she declares. "For my age, I'm in good health except for a few things that cannot be corrected. If anything *can* be corrected, I'll go do it."

That was the attitude Jeanette was armed with in 1990 when, at the age of 86, she began feeling jolts of pain throughout her lower left jaw. After examining the troubled area, her family dentist announced that her first bicuspid on that side had fractured and would have to be extracted. There was more bad news: advanced decay was imperiling the third molar. Since those two teeth served as the anchors for a five-unit permanent bridge, some major redesign of her teeth on that side would be required.

Jeanette already had reason to grumble about a removable four-unit bridge she was wearing on her upper right side. It felt fine—once it was in position. But taking it out every night and reinstalling it every morning confounded the octogenarian. "It was hard for me, and I can't quite say why," she says. "The bridge had some little edge to it that you had to get into the right place. I just did not like it."

Confronted with the additional problems, Jeanette was intrigued when her doctor mentioned that implants might be a solution. "I had heard about them, but I didn't know if my jawbone and gums would be in good enough condition to allow me to get them," she remembers.

> **Jeanette Silber:**
>
> *Sometimes I look at myself in the mirror, all dressed up, and I think, Oh boy, I'm not worth all that money. But I never felt that way about my implants. I am really delighted with them. They feel just like my own teeth. I never think they're not mine.*

In order to assess the state of her bone and gums, x-rays were taken. The results were unequivocal: both the quantity and quality of her bone was good.

As soon as Jeanette heard the news, she beamed and posed a question. Could she replace her troublesome partial denture, a four-unit removable upper bridge, with implants at the same time that she received four implants in her lower jaw? Informed that there was no reason not to do this, her response was immediate. "Give me the first date you've got!" she directed.

Her friends had a very different reaction when she told them what she was about to do. "Oh my, they all thought I was crazy. They said they would never spend that amount of money at their age." But that kind of thinking didn't make sense to Jeanette. "If I wanted to buy a car, I would buy a car," she mused. "I'm important to myself. I feel, you have to take care of yourself. Nobody else does."

She also brushed aside any worries that the surgery might hurt. "The doctor gave me pills in case I had pain that night, but I never took one." Despite having extractions and seven implants placed, "I didn't have any pain," she states.

Not long after her 99th birthday, Jeanette reflected on her longevity. She couldn't credit exercise, she declared. "I haven't played golf since I was 50. And it's certainly not my diet. I'm a *very* small eater, but what I love most in the world are desserts. I could eat sweets all day long, and never miss anything else. I never eat breakfast. At noon I may eat cereal, and then I have a decent dinner. But I really live on sweets. I could take a handful of candy three times a day."

"I think it must be genes," she admits. "My mother lived to be 91 1/2; my father was 88 when he died. They were married 68 years." Jeanette and her husband, who died more than 25 years ago, never had children, but she describes with pride her wide circle of loving relatives and friends.

Many of those friends are losing teeth, "and yet they won't spend the money to get implants." She sounds frustrated by this resistance. There were times, she recounts, when she has been all dressed up to go out to some charity gala. "Sometimes I look at myself in the mirror and sort of price what I have on, and I think, 'Oh boy, I'm not worth all that money!'"

But she has never felt that way about her implants, she asserts. "I am really delighted with them. They feel just like my own teeth. I never think that they're not mine."

Glossary

Abutment: A metal post attached to the implant and projecting through the gum tissue; the final tooth restoration attaches to the abutment.

Anesthesia: A drug-induced loss of sensation; may be local (e.g., Novocain); incomplete (as in "twilight" sedation); or complete (general anesthesia).

Appliance: A dental device that replaces missing teeth.

Bridge: A prosthetic appliance that rests on the adjacent teeth and suspends a dummy tooth or teeth between them. A bridge may be removable by the patient or cemented into place.

Bruxism: Clenching or grinding the teeth; common during sleep (nocturnal bruxism).

Cap: A restoration that is cemented over the majority or the entire crown of a tooth; also called a crown.

Contraindication: A condition that makes a particular treatment inadvisable.

Crown: See cap.

Dental implant: A metal replacement for a tooth root. It forms a secure foundation for the replacement tooth (prosthesis). It may be placed in the bone (endosseous), on the bone (subperiosteal), or through the bone (transosteal).

Endosseous: In the bone; endosseous dental implants are those placed into the jawbone, with which they fuse.

Flipper: A removable temporary prosthesis that usually replaces one tooth.

Gingivitis: The early stage of periodontal disease, which may result in puffy, tender, bleeding gums.

Growth factor: A substance in the platelets of blood that helps to regenerate and heal bone and gum tissue.

Osseointegration: From the words "osseo," meaning bone and "integrate," meaning to unite; this term refers to the process in which the implant fuses to the jawbone.

Panorex: An x-ray taken outside the mouth that provides a panoramic view of the interior of the mouth and surrounding anatomy (e.g., sinuses, jawbone nerve pathways).

Periapical: A localized x-ray view of one to three teeth.

Periodontics: The dental specialty of treating bone and the hard and soft tissues of the mouth; the practitioner is called a periodontist.

Periodontitis: A disease state that affects the surrounding and supporting structures of the teeth such as gum tissue and jawbone; commonly called periodontal disease.

Platelet-rich plasma: A substance processed from the patient's own blood at the time of surgery. The processing concentrates the blood platelets, which contain huge amounts of growth and wound-healing factors. Platelet-rich plasma is used to improve healing of the bone and gum tissue.

Prosthesis: A dental appliance incorporating teeth; examples include a crown, cap, bridge, denture; also called a restoration. A prosthesis may be removable by the patient, removable by the doctor, or cemented into place.

Prosthodontics: The dental specialty of making crowns, bridges, dentures, and other prostheses; the practitioner is called a prosthodontist.

Provisional: Any treatment that is temporary; e.g. a provisional denture or implant.

Restore: To attach a prosthesis.

Restoration: See prosthesis.

Socket: The defect in the jawbone remaining after the removal of a tooth.

Soft tissue: The inner cheeks and inner aspect of the lips, floor of the mouth, tongue, hard and soft palates, and gums.

Subperiosteal: Below the gum; a subperiosteal dental implant is one placed beneath the gum tissue and on top of the jawbone.

Titanium: A strong, lightweight metallic element that is extremely resistant to corrosion; the most popular metal used in dental and many orthopedic implants.

Transosteal: Through the bone; a transosteal dental implant is inserted via an incision under the chin and placed through the front of the lower jawbone.

Appendix A
Joann Platman:
One Patient's Testimonial

I can remember the first time dental implants were shown on national television. It was a story on the evening news. Peter Jennings narrated a segment about this "new" dental technique showing actual implants placed in a patient's mouth. I can still see the pained look on Peter Jennings' face when the segment ended. Yes, it did look "bionic-like," but I saw it as a vision into the future.

I had been wearing dentures for almost nine years and had resigned myself to accepting this as my lot in life. I was not a bad person, but somehow this awful event had happened to me. It is humbling and emotionally devastating to face this reality. Denture-wearing was the brunt of jokes and a sign of advancing age. It was a real failure in my life. I could have a job. I could be loved by my family, but my feelings of self-worth would never allow me to fully enjoy what is normal for most people. I don't think anyone knows how difficult it can be to lose your dignity in this manner. Having implants offered me a second chance.

What follows is my perspective as an actual patient having gone through this procedure.

From my point of view, I wanted to have my implants done by the best-qualified people out there. I know that I was very lucky to have Dr. Charles Babbush and Dr. Evan Tetelman. I trusted them, and they showed me they cared about me, which I think made the many, many visits involved with having the procedure done bearable. Make no mistake: this is not a decision to take lightly. It takes courage to undergo all that is involved and resolve to see it to the end. You are going to spend a lot of time in the dentist's chair and make frequent visits to the surgeon to check on your progress. Also, there is the financial investment, which is significant. I had been told to equate having implants with buying a luxury car but with the added advantage of knowing they will last a lifetime. I guess that means that my smile can be compared to driving a BMW!

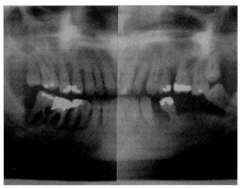

Figure AP.1 The x-ray from the initial contact with the patient in 1990 shows advanced decay and periodontal disease of her entire mouth.

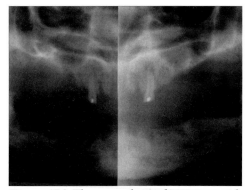

Figure AP.2 The x-ray shows the patient with only two teeth remaining in the upper jaw in 1998.

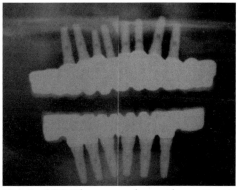

Figure AP.3 The x-ray shows the patient's mouth after reconstruction with implants.

I did have extensive work done. I needed eight implants in the upper and six implants in the lower jaw. First, I had a CAT scan to determine if there was enough bone remaining in my mouth to support all the implants. Luckily this was the case, and a computerized model was made of my mouth showing where the implants would be positioned. I could visually see what was going to happen, but I did not know the reality of what was to occur.

All the implants were placed in one visit at the surgeon's office under twilight sedation. In addition, I was given shots of Novocain, which helped to relieve the pain while those implants were placed. I went home exhausted and relieved that the surgery was over. I had a painkiller prescription to use if needed, along with instructions to apply ice packs to my face to help with the swelling.

Actually, in the days following the surgery, there was not much pain. However, I did start showing bruising on the second day, and by the third day, I had two black eyes and some swelling. I had not expected that I would bruise to the extent I did. The bruises and swelling did fade within a week or two, but I had some numbness in my lower jaw.

> **Joann Platman:**
>
> *I feel the best I have ever felt about myself. The results are truly amazing. My smile is more than I could have hoped for, and I smile all the time. I also enjoy foods again that I never thought would be possible.*
>
> *All of this could not have happened if it weren't for the skill and persistence of all those professionals involved who made sure everything was done just right. I will always remain grateful to them for their combined efforts.*

Once I was able to return to my normal routine of working and going out in public, I felt better physically and mentally. The healing stage then began. The dentures were fitted over my implants, and I was able to eat and speak as before implant surgery.

After four months, the second surgery was performed to uncover the implants, and healing caps were placed. This was done with a local anesthetic, but I was given nitrous oxide to help me relax. This surgery was relatively pain-free, and I was back at work the next day. Also, I am happy to say that the numbness in my lower jaw did go away over time, although I had some concern over how long this feeling would last.

Two-hour visits to the dentist were the norm. At each visit, caps were removed and measurements taken in order to have the appliances made. Each visit was a step closer to the finish. That's what kept me going.

I chose to have non-removable appliances, which are secured by screws and can only be removed by the dentist. This is what I had wanted from very early on when I was still learning about all the possibilities. The actual final visit with everything fitted and placed in my mouth took place approximately ten months after my first surgery. I have been told this is excellent. It could have taken longer. After that final screw was tightened to hold the appliances in place, I could not believe that there was total stability in my mouth. The feeling was incredible. I had not had that feeling for a long, long time. I talked out loud a lot at first to become accustomed to what was a new, yet familiar feeling inside my mouth. It really did not take more than a week or so to become fully comfortable and at ease speaking and eating. Cleaning took on a whole new meaning. It was a little tricky learning to get around with all my new cleaning tools, but that too got easier and I now feel quite comfortable negotiating around and through the appliances.

It has been several years since the surgery (February 1999) and the work was completed (October 1999). I feel the best I have ever felt about myself. The results are truly amazing. My smile is more than I could have hoped for, and I smile all the time. I also enjoy foods again that I never thought would be possible. All of this could not have happened if it weren't for the skill and persistence of all those professionals involved who made sure everything was done just right. I will always remain grateful to them for their combined efforts and to my husband, who endured everything with me and encouraged me from day one and always loved me no matter what.

Finally, implants are not an easy road to travel, but if you do choose to make that journey, you will feel like you have been given an incredible gift. I know I have.

Appendix B:
Resources

Dental Associations

Academy of General Dentistry
211 E. Chicago Ave.
Chicago, IL 60611
Phone: (312) 440-4300
E-mail: adg.org

**American Academy of
Cosmetic Dentistry**
5401 World Dairy Dr.
Madison, WI 53718
Phone: (800) 543-9220
www.aacc.com

**American Academy of Esthetic
Dentistry**
401 N. Michigan Ave.
Chicago, IL 60611
Phone: (312) 321-5121
www.estheticacademy.org

**American Association of Oral
and Maxillofacial Surgeons**
9700 W. Bryn Mawr Ave.
Rosemont, IL 60018
Phone: (800) 822-6637
Fax: (847) 678-6286
www.aaoms.org

**American Academy of
Periodontology**
737 N. Michigan Ave., Ste. 800
Chicago, IL 60611
Phone: (312) 787-5518
www.perio.org

**American College of
Prosthodontists**
211 East Chicago Ave.,
Ste. 1000
Chicago, IL 60611
Phone: (312) 573-1260
Fax: (312) 573-1257
www.prosthodontics.org

American Dental Association
211 E. Chicago Ave.
Chicago, IL 60611
Phone: (312) 440-2500
Fax: (312) 440-7494
www.ada.org

American Dental Hygienists'
Association
444 N. Michigan Ave., Ste. 3400
Chicago, IL 60611
Phone: (312) 440-8900
www.adha.org

Implant Organizations

Academy of Osseointegration
85 W. Algonquin Rd., Ste. 550
Arlington Heights, IL 60005
Phone: (800) 656-7736
Fax: (847) 439-1569
E-mail: foundation@osseo.org

**American Academy of Implant
Dentistry**
211 East Chicago Ave., Ste. 750
Chicago, IL 60611
Phone: (312) 335-155-
Fax: (312) 335-9090
www.aaid@aaid-implant.org

**Institute for Dental Implant
Awareness**
11601 Wilshire Blvd., Ste. 500
Los Angeles, CA 90025
Phone: (800) 936-4342
www.dentalimplants.org

**International Congress of Oral
Implantologists**
248 Lorraine Ave., Third Floor
Upper Montclair, NJ 07043-
1454
Phone: (973) 783-6300
Fax: (973) 783-1175
Email: icoi@dentalimplants.com

Implant Companies

3i Implant Innovations
4555 Riverside Dr.
Palm Beach Gardens, FL 33410
Phone: (800) 342-5454
Fax: (561) 776-1272
www.3i-online.com

Ace Surgical Supply Co.
P.O. Box 1710
Brockton, MA 02303
Phone: (800) 441-3100
Fax: (800) 583-3150
E-Mail: info@acesurgical.com
www.acesurgical.com

**Altiva Natural Tooth
Replacement System**
9800 Southern Pines Blvd., Ste. I
Charlotte, NC
Phone: (866) 425-8482
Fax: (704) 409-1771
www.altivacorp.com

Astra
430 Bedford St.
Lexington, MA
Phone: (800) 531-3481
Fax: (781) 861-7787
www.astratechusa.com

Biocon, Inc.
501 Arborway
Boston, MA 02130
Phone: (800) 88-BICON
Fax: (800) 28-BICON
E-Mail: bicon@bicon.com
www.bicon.com

BioHorizons
One Perimeter Park S., Ste. 230
South Birmingham, AL
Phone: (888) 246-8338
Fax: (205) 88870-0304
E-Mail: info@biohorizons.de
www. biohorizons.com

Centerpulse Dental
1900 Aston Ave.
Carlsbad, CA 92008
Phone: (800) 854-7019
Fax: (760) 431-7811
www.centerpulse-dental.com

Dentatus
Jakobsdalssvagen 14-16
S-126 Hagersten
Phone, USA: (800) 323-3136
Phone: +46 (8) 54 65 09 40
Fax: +46 (8) 54 65 09 01
E-Mail: info@dentatus.se
www.dentatus.com

Friadent CeraMed
A division of Dentsply
International
12860 W. Cedar Dr., Ste. 110
Lakewood, CO 80228
Phone: (800) 426-7836
www.dentsplyfc.com

Imtec Europe GmbH
Industriepark Hochst, F821
65926 Frankfurt am Main
Phone: 0-800-46832-000
Fax: (069) 305 444 56
E-Mail: europe@imtec.com
www.imtec.com

**Interphase Implants Inc./
Smooth Staple**
19928 Farmington Rd.
Livonia, MI 48152
Phone: (248) 442-1460
Fax: (248) 477-4338
E-mail: interpha@mich.com

Lifecore
3515 Lyman Blvd.
Chaska, MN 55318
Phone: (800) 752-2663
Fax: (952) 368-4324
www.lifecore.com

Nobel Biocare
22715 Savi Ranch Pkwy.
Yorba Linda, CA 92887
Phone: (800) 322-5001
Fax: (714) 998-9236
www.nobelbiocareusa.com

**Oraltronics
Dental Implant Technology
GmbH**
Herrlichkeit 4 – D – 288199
Bremen, Germany
Phone: ++49-(0) 421-43939-0
Fax: ++49-(0) 421-443936
E-Mail: info@oraltronics.com
www.oraltronics.com

Park Dental Research
19 W. 34th St.
New York, NY 10001
Phone: (800) 243-7372
Fax: (212) 268-6845
www.parkdental.com

Straumann Implant Co.
Reservoir Place
1601 Trapelo Rd.
Waltham, MA 02451
Phone: (800) 449-8168
Fax: (781) 890-6464
E-mail: info.usa@straumann.com
www.straumann.com

TMI Inc.
882 E. Coast Dr.
Atlantic Beach, FL 32233
Phone: (800) 401-3647
www.boskermi.com

Valley Dental Arts
1745 Northwester Ave.
Stillwater, MN 55082
Phone: (800) 328-9157
www.valleydentalarts.com

Biotechnology Companies

Friadent CeraMed
A division of Dentsply
International
12860 W. Cedar Dr., Ste. 110
Lakewood, CO 80228
Phone: (800) 426-7836
www.dentsplyfc.com

GenSci Orthobiologics Inc.
2 Goodyear Dr.
Irvine, CA 92618
Phone: (949) 855-7129
Fax: (949) 595-8705
www.gensciinc.com

Harvest Technologies Corp.
40 Grissom Rd.
Plymouth, MA 02360
Phone: (508) 732-7500
Fax: (508) 732-0400
www.harvesttech.com

**Materialise NV/Columbia
Scientific**
810-X Cromwell Park Dr.
Glen Burnie, MD 21061
Phone: (888) 327-8202
Fax: (443) 557-0036
www.simplant@materialise.com

Salvin Dental Specialties
3450 Latrobe Dr.
Charlotte, NC 28211
Phone: (800) 535-6566
Fax: (704) 442-5424
www.salvin.com

The Amara Institute
P.O. Box 367
Stillwater, MN 55082
Phone: (877) 520-0791
www.theamarainstitute.com

Appendix C
Credits

The author gratefully acknowledges the sources of the following illustrations.

0.2 Elsevier Sciences USA (St. Louis)

1.1 Harvard University Press (Boston) and Nature

1.2 Musée du Louvre (Paris, France)

1.3 Musée de l'École Dentaire de Paris (Paris, France)

1.4 Peabody Museum, Harvard University (Boston)

1.5 Pennsylvania Academy of the Fine Arts (Philadelphia)

1.6 Museum of Fine Arts (Boston) and the National Portrait Gallery, Smithsonian Institute (Washington, D.C.)

1.7 Case Western Reserve University, School of Dentistry (Cleveland)

1.12 A-D Elsevier Sciences USA (St. Louis)

1.13 A-H Elsevier Sciences USA (St. Louis)

2.4C Elsevier Sciences USA (St. Louis)

4.8 Elsevier Sciences USA (St. Louis)

6.7A,B Dr. Paul Petrungaro

Index